Fast Facts for Healthcare
Professionals

Dermatoses in Skin of Color

Paul Devakar Yesudian MRCP MD DipNB
Consultant Dermatologist
Wrexham Maelor Hospital
Wrexham, UK

Patrick Yesudian FRCP
Consultant Dermatologist
Retired Professor of Dermatology
Madras Medical College
Chennai, India

Rohan Isaac Yesudian BA
Medical student
School of Clinical Medicine
University of Cambridge
Cambridge, UK

Declaration of Independence
This book is as balanced and as practical as we can make it.
Ideas for improvement are always welcome: fastfacts@karger.com

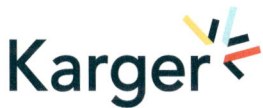

HEALTHCARE

Fast Facts: Dermatoses in Skin of Color
First published 2025

Text © 2025 Paul Devakar Yesudian, Patrick Yesudian, Rohan Isaac Yesudian
© 2025 in this edition S. Karger Publishers Limited

S. Karger Publishers Limited, Merchant House, 5 East St. Helen Street, Abingdon, Oxford OX14 5EG, UK

Book orders can be placed by telephone or email, or via the website.
Please telephone +41 61 306 1440 or email orders@karger.com
To order via the website, please go to karger.com

Fast Facts is a trademark of S. Karger Publishers Limited.

All rights reserved. No part of this publication may be reproduced, stored in a retrieval system, or transmitted in any form or by any means, electronic, mechanical, photocopying, recording, or otherwise, without the express permission of the publisher.

The rights of Paul Devakar Yesudian, Patrick Yesudian, and Rohan Isaac Yesudian to be identified as the authors of this work have been asserted in accordance with the Copyright, Designs & Patents Act 1988 Sections 77 and 78.

The publisher and the authors have made every effort to ensure the accuracy of this book, but cannot accept responsibility for any errors or omissions.

For all drugs, please consult the product labeling approved in your country for prescribing information.

Registered names, trademarks, etc. used in this book, even when not marked as such, are not to be considered unprotected by law.

A CIP record for this title is available from the British Library.

ISBN: 978-3-318-07287-7

Yesudian PD (Paul Devakar)
Fast Facts: Dermatoses in Skin of Color/
Paul Devakar Yesudian, Patrick Yesudian, Rohan Isaac Yesudian

Typesetting by Amnet, Chennai, India.
Printed in the UK with Xpedient Print.

List of abbreviations	5
Introduction	7
Differential diagnoses by history and clinical features	9
Refining the differential diagnosis with investigations and tests	57
Presentation and management of common dermatoses in skin of color	71
Presentation and management of dermatoses predominantly seen in skin of color	93
Useful resources	123
Index	125

List of abbreviations

ACE: angiotensin-converting enzyme

AIDS: acquired immunodeficiency syndrome

ALP: actinic lichen planus

BCC: basal cell carcinoma

CNS: central nervous system

CO_2: carbon dioxide

COFS (syndrome): cerebro-oculo-facial-skeletal

COVID-19: coronavirus disease 2019

CT: computed tomography

CTCL: cutaneous T-cell lymphoma

DCPA: dermatitis cruris pustulosa et atrophicans

DRESS (syndrome): drug reaction with eosinophilia and systemic symptoms

EO: exogenous ochronosis

HIV: human immunodeficiency virus

HS: hidradenitis suppurativa

Ig: immunoglobulin

IL: interleukin

LEOPARD (syndrome): lentigenes, electrocardiographic conduction defects, ocular hypertelorism, pulmonary stenosis, abnormalities of the genitals, retarded growth, deafness

LP: lichen planus

LPP: lichen planus pigmentosus

MF: mycosis fungoides

MRI: magnetic resonance imaging

PAPA (syndrome): pyogenic arthritis, pyoderma gangrenosum, and acne

PCOS: polycystic ovary syndrome

PFB: pseudofolliculitis barbae

PIH: post-inflammatory hyperpigmentation

PKDL: post-kala-azar dermal leishmaniasis

PLEVA: pityriasis lichenoides et varioliformis acuta

POEMS (syndrome): polyneuropathy, organomegaly, endocrinopathy, monoclonal plasma cell disorder, skin changes

PUVA: psoralen plus ultraviolet A (phototherapy)

SAPHO (syndrome): synovitis, acne, pustulosis, hyperostosis, osteitis

SCC: squamous cell carcinoma

SOC: skin of color

TNF: tumor necrosis factor

UV: ultraviolet

VDRL: Venereal Disease Research Laboratory (blood test)

YAG: yttrium-aluminum-garnett

Introduction

For those practicing dermatology among people of White ethnicity, dermatoses in skin of color (SOC) can appear puzzling. It is difficult to know whether the different appearance of skin lesions in SOC is due to genetic or socioeconomic factors, or if it is the dark color of the skin causing the variation.

Even though skin conditions affect people of all skin types, the vast majority of dermatological research has been conducted on those with lighter skin tones, leaving people with SOC, that is, those of African, Asian, Native American, Middle Eastern, and Hispanic descent, without adequate representation or understanding of their unique skin condition.

Having worked as a resident in dermatology after graduating from the Madras Medical College in the late 1950s, I was reasonably conversant with the diagnoses of common skin diseases like psoriasis, lichen planus, tinea, and eczema in South Indian patients who are, on average, of darker hue (Fitzpatrick type IV and V). Then I went to the UK for postgraduate training and to my utter consternation I struggled to get 10% of the diagnoses correct simply because of the skin color, or rather the lack of it, of a predominantly White population of British patients. After a few months my eyes and brain got used to assessing signs and symptoms in this new situation. Conversely, a few decades later when my senior consultant from Scotland visited my department in Madras, he found it difficult to recognize common dermatoses on SOC.

Given the ease of travel between countries nowadays and the large number of global migrants, a dermatologist of any nationality may encounter dermatoses among patients of color. There are also certain dermatoses that occur almost exclusively in SOC, such as dermatosis papulosa nigra, dermatitis cruris pustulosa et atrophicans, and disseminated infundibulofolliculitis, with which dermatologists practicing in European countries should familiarize themselves for better patient care.

Adding further complexity to the diagnosis of dermatoses in SOC has been the increasingly popular global trend for skin lightening. The desire to look 'fair' has led to overuse of bleaching preparations containing mercury and hydroquinone, which not only cause skin disfigurement in the form of acquired ochronosis but, rarely, general medical problems like kidney damage. While some countries (for example, Kenya) have banned the manufacture and sale of whitening products, skin bleaching is widely practiced elsewhere, including the USA, South East Asia, and India, and has become a billion-dollar industry.

So, why another book on dermatology? We believe that this book is different since it brings to the fore the number of variables in morphology in SOC, resulting in a long shopping list of differential diagnoses, which will serve as a ready reckoner for students, registrars, postgraduates, nurses, and general practitioners who are likely to encounter patients of color. Drawing on the latest scientific research and clinical expertise, we aim to shed light on the incidence, presentation, and treatment of dermatoses in SOC, for a patient population who have historically been underserved by the medical community.

Professor Patrick Yesudian

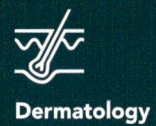

Dermatology

1 Differential diagnoses by history and clinical features

Dermatological symptoms
  1.1 Itching without rash *10*
  1.2 Hyperhidrosis *11*
  1.3 Fever and rash *13*
Abnormal pigmentation
  1.4 Generalized hyperpigmentation *14*
  1.5 White patches on face *16*
  1.6 Linear hypopigmentation *17*
  1.7 Palmar pigmentation *18*
  1.8 Reticulate acropigmentation *19*
  1.9 Oral pigmentation *20*
  1.10 Pigmented tumors *21*
Bumps, blisters, and pustules
  1.11 Comedones *22*
  1.12 Warty/verrucous dermatoses *22*
  1.13 Infantile blisters *23*
  1.14 Sterile pustules *25*
  1.15 Palmoplantar pustules *26*
Lesions with a characteristic shape
  1.16 Umbilicated lesions *27*
  1.17 Serpiginous lesions *28*
  1.18 Annular lesions *29*
Dermatoses with a specific pattern or distribution
  1.19 Migratory dermatoses *30*
  1.20 Linear morphology *31*
  1.21 Digitate dermatoses *32*
  1.22 Christmas-tree pattern *33*
  1.23 Sporotrichoid distribution *34*
  1.24 Zosteriform/blaschkoid dermatoses *35*
Pathergy
  1.25 Pathergy *36*
Perforating disorders
  1.26a Primary perforating disorders *37*
  1.26b Secondary perforating disorders *37*
Skin conditions masquerading as common dermatoses
  1.27 Lichenoid dermatoses *38*
  1.28 Psoriasiform dermatoses *39*
  1.29 Acneiform dermatoses *40*
  1.30 Pellagra-like dermatoses *41*
  1.31 Varioliform scarring *42*
  1.32 Photosensitive disorders in children *43*
Dermatoses of the face and ears
  1.33 Leonine facies *44*
  1.34 Destructive nasal lesions *45*
  1.35 Loss of the lateral one-third of the eyebrows *46*
  1.36 Thickened pinnae *46*
Dermatoses of the nails and palms
  1.37 Pseudo-Hutchinson sign *47*
  1.38 Koilonychia *48*
  1.39 Nail pitting *49*
  1.40 Palmar pits *50*

HEALTHCARE

More than 3000 skin diseases have been described worldwide, affecting nearly 2 billion people.[1,2] However, dermatologists are often in short supply, particularly in rural areas, and initial diagnosis often falls to non-specialists with limited equipment and/or specialist knowledge on cutaneous disorders. Careful history-taking and examination of patients helps elicit the key symptoms and signs of skin conditions, providing clinicians with useful differential diagnoses to guide further workup and treatment decisions.

Observing a patient's demeanor and distress levels allows fuller understanding beyond the visible dermatosis, potentially warranting examination of unaffected areas. The goal is to attain sufficient information about the condition to optimize its management. In many instances, clinicians may not need to achieve diagnostic certainty before initiating treatment, particularly if the conditions in the differential diagnosis share similar initial treatment. For example, an inflammatory lesion may indicate contact dermatitis or psoriasis, both of which can be initially treated with topical corticosteroids.

Here, we provide a list of etiologies for a wide range of dermatological signs and symptoms for patients with skin of color (SOC).

Dermatological symptoms

1.1 Itching without rash. Itchy skin (pruritus) in the absence of a rash is common and has many causes. It can be generalized or localized and may be an important symptom of systemic conditions.[3]

Inflammatory. Atopic eczema, xerosis, urticaria, dermatitis herpetiformis (Figure 1.1), systemic lupus erythematosus, dermatomyositis, pre-bullous pemphigoid.

Infections. Scabies, parasitic infections, HIV infection.

Medical conditions. Kidney disease, liver disease (cholestatic), iron deficiency, malabsorption.

Endocrine. Hypothyroidism, hyperthyroidism, hyperparathyroidism, diabetes mellitus.

Neoplasms. Lymphoma, invisible mycosis fungoides, mastocytosis, carcinoid tumors, polycythemia vera, CNS tumors, hypereosinophilic syndrome, solid tumors of the cervix, prostate, or colon.

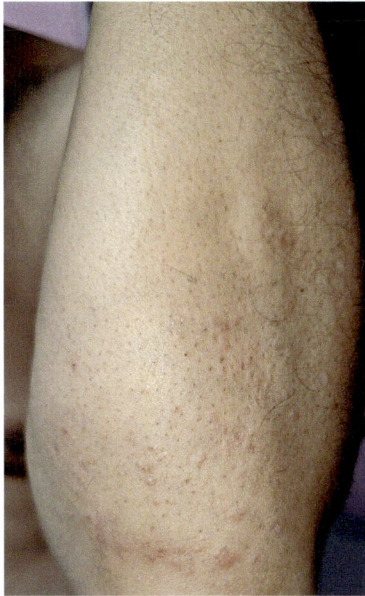 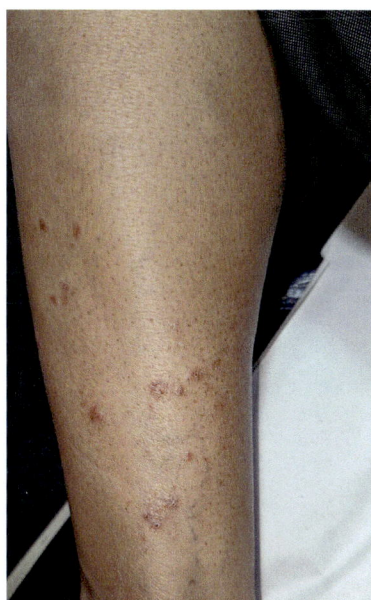

Figure 1.1 Dermatitis herpetiformis is an intensely itchy condition caused by gluten sensitivity. The rash can appear as non-specific erythematous papules, and sometimes the skin may appear normal.

Neuropathic. Brachioradial pruritus, notalgia paresthetica, post-herpetic neuralgia, vulvodynia, multiple sclerosis.

Drug-related

Recreational drugs. Cocaine.

Prescribed medications. Opioids, angiotensin-converting enzyme (ACE) inhibitors, amiodarone, estrogens, statins, allopurinol.

Other. Pregnancy, psychogenic pruritus, perimenopausal symptoms, aquagenic pruritus.

1.2 Hyperhidrosis is excessive sweating in the absence of a heat stimulus. It can be localized or generalized and have primary (more common) or secondary causes.[4]

Generalized hyperhidrosis, that is, excessive sweating that affects the whole body, has various etiologies.

Physiological. Fever, reaction to spicy food, menopause, pregnancy, obesity.

Inflammatory. Sarcoidosis, rheumatoid arthritis.

Infections. Acute bacterial and viral infections, tuberculosis (Figure 1.2), brucellosis, malaria, post-encephalitis, tabes dorsalis, HIV infection.

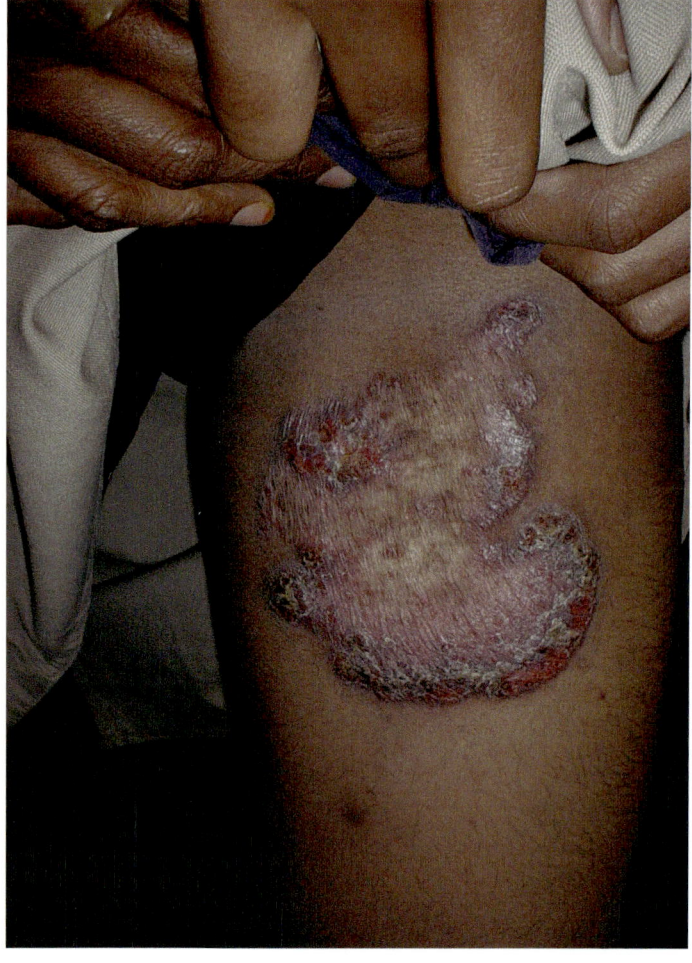

Figure 1.2 Lupus vulgaris associated with pulmonary tuberculosis. Profuse night sweats are a dominant symptom of tuberculosis.

Medical conditions. Cardiovascular failure, respiratory failure.
 Endocrine. Hyperthyroidism, diabetes mellitus, diabetes insipidus, acromegaly, pheochromocytoma, hyperpituitarism, carcinoid tumors or disease, hypoglycemia.
 Neurological. Parkinson's disease, post-sympathectomy, cortical (central) hyperhidrosis, familial dysautonomia.
 Neoplasms. Lymphoma, myeloproliferative disorders.
 Genetic. Congenital autonomic dysfunction associated with pain loss, porphyria, POEMS syndrome, phenylketonuria.
 Drug-related. Cholinesterase inhibitors, tricyclic antidepressants, nicotinamide, alcohol, recreational drugs, meperidine, propranolol.
 Other. Cold injury.
 Localized hyperhidrosis affects one or more body areas, most commonly the armpits, palms, soles, and/or face.
 Physiological. Anxiety, primary craniofacial hyperhidrosis.
 Neurological. Auriculotemporal syndrome (Frey's syndrome), CNS tumor or disease, spinal injury, syringomyelia, peripheral neuropathy, stroke, Grierson–Gopalan syndrome, complex partial pain syndrome (reflex sympathetic dystrophy).

1.3 Fever and rash. A combination of fever and rash may potentially indicate sinister underlying causes that need to be ruled out.[5]
 Inflammatory. Systemic lupus erythematosus (Figure 1.3), pustular psoriasis, Sweet's syndrome (acute febrile neutrophilic dermatosis), Kawasaki disease, dermatomyositis, erythema multiforme, sarcoidosis.
 Infections. Dengue (Dengue fever), viral infections (varicella-zoster [chickenpox], parvovirus B19, rubella [German measles], enterovirus, herpes simplex, HIV), scarlet fever, toxic shock syndrome, secondary syphilis, meningococcemia, endocarditis, leptospirosis.
 Neoplasms. Lymphoma.
 Drug-related. DRESS syndrome.

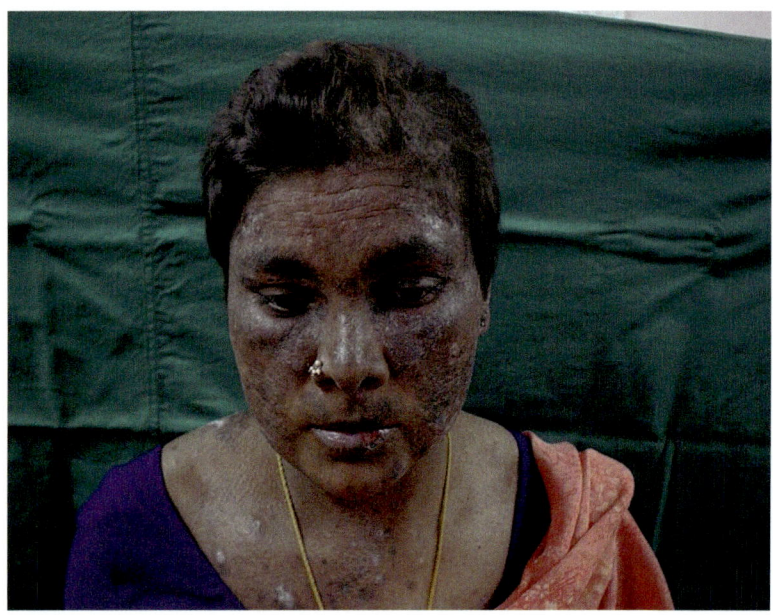

Figure 1.3 Severe systemic lupus erythematosus, an autoimmune disease that causes widespread inflammation and tissue damage.

Abnormal pigmentation

1.4 Generalized hyperpigmentation can be multifactorial in origin. It can be inherited or acquired, and a systemic or cutaneous cause needs to be ascertained.[6,7]

Inflammatory. Lichen planus pigmentosus, post-inflammatory pigmentation, erythema dyschromicum perstans (ashy dermatosis), progressive systemic sclerosis, eczema.

Infections. HIV/AIDS, visceral leishmaniasis, malaria.

Metabolic. B12 deficiency, pellagra.

Endocrine. Addison's disease, adrenoleukodystrophy, congenital adrenal hyperplasia, hyperthyroidism, Nelson's syndrome, diabetes mellitus, primary pigmented nodular adrenocortical disease.

Medical conditions. Liver failure, kidney failure, cachexia, protein deficiency, malabsorption, primary biliary cirrhosis, porphyria cutanea tarda, Whipple's disease.

Neoplasms. Carcinoid syndrome, metastatic melanoma, mycosis fungoides, ectopic adrenocorticotropic hormone-secreting tumor, pheochromocytoma.

Genetic. Cronkhite–Canada syndrome, dyschromatosis universalis hereditaria, Niemann–Pick disease, Gaucher's disease, Schimke immuno-osseous dysplasia, POEMS syndrome, Wilson's disease, xeroderma pigmentosum, neurofibromatosis (Figure 1.4).

Drug-related. Amiodarone, antimalarials, minocycline, clofazimine, heavy metals (gold, bismuth, silver, arsenic), hydroxyurea, imipramine, bleomycin.

Other. Ultraviolet (UV) radiation, carbon baby syndrome (acquired universal melanosis), pregnancy, bronze baby syndrome, eosinophilia–myalgia syndrome, hemochromatosis, familial diffuse hypermelanosis, toxic oil syndrome.

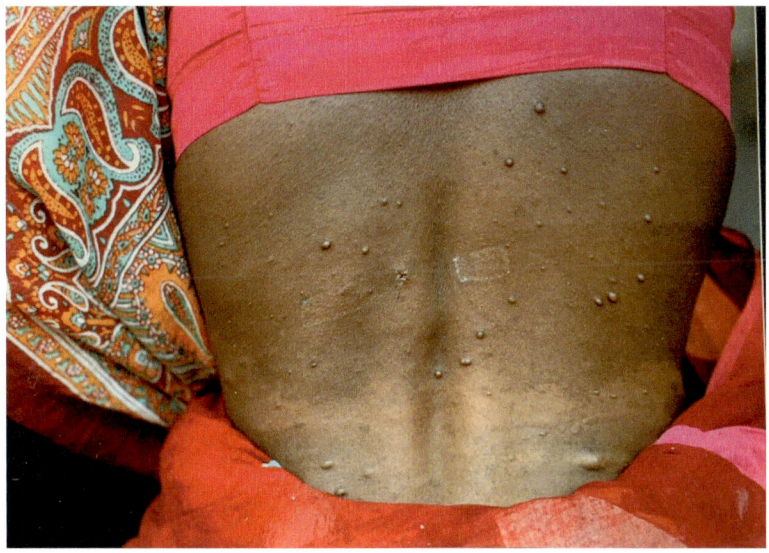

Figure 1.4 Generalized hyperpigmentation on the back of a patient with neurofibromatosis. Normal skin can be seen near the waistband.

1.5 White patches on face. Although hypopigmentation on the face is most often asymptomatic and is generally benign, rarely it can be caused by serious and, sometimes, disabling conditions.[8,9] White patches on the face are more noticeable in people with darker skin, and, in some instances, can result in stigma, affecting confidence in work and home lives.

Inflammatory. Pityriasis alba, vitiligo, post-inflammatory hypopigmentation, extragenital lichen sclerosus, sarcoidosis, polymorphic light eruption (Figure 1.5).

Infections. Leprosy (Hansen's disease), pityriasis versicolor, secondary syphilis, yaws, post-kala-azar dermal leishmaniasis (PKDL), pinta, onchocerciasis.

Neoplasms. Hypopigmented mycosis fungoides.

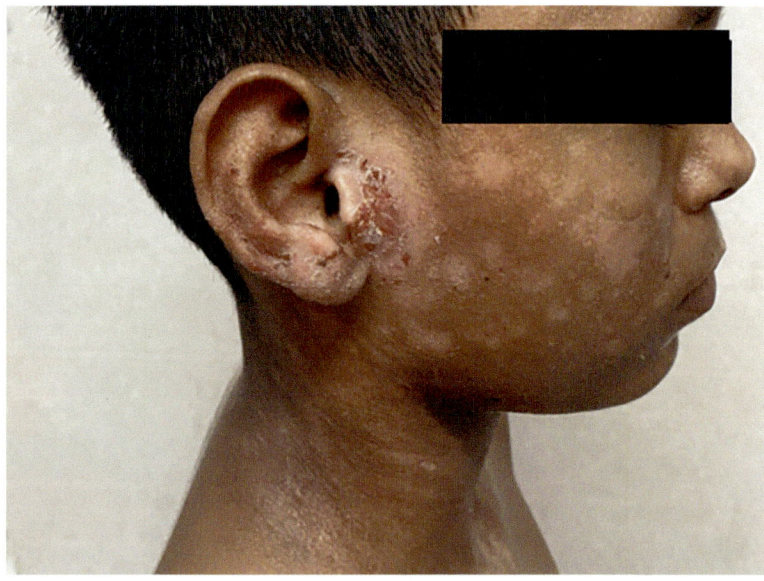

Figure 1.5 Polymorphic light eruption, a delayed hypersensitivity reaction to ultraviolet light.

Genetic. Ash-leaf macule, nevus of Ito, albinism, piebaldism, Waardenburg syndrome, homocystinuria, nevus anemicus, nevus depigmentosus.

Drug- and chemical-related. Intralesional and topical corticosteroids, diphenylcyclopropenone (for alopecia areata), arsenic, phenols, benzene derivatives (used as antiseptics).

Other. Halo nevi, scars.

1.6 Linear hypopigmentation. There are multiple causes of reduced skin color that present in a linear distribution. Certain dermatoses may be restricted to Blaschko's lines, which are the embryological pathways for epidermal cell migration.[10,11]

Inflammatory. Lichen striatus (Figure 1.6), post-inflammatory hypopigmentation, segmental vitiligo, lichen sclerosus, pityriasis alba, linear lichen nitidus, white dermographism, linear morphea.

Congenital. Epidermal nevus, incontinentia pigmenti (stage IV), hypomelanosis of Ito, focal dermal hypoplasia (Goltz syndrome), nevus depigmentosus, Menkes' kinky-hair disease (female carrier), segmental ash-leaf macule, linear piebaldism.

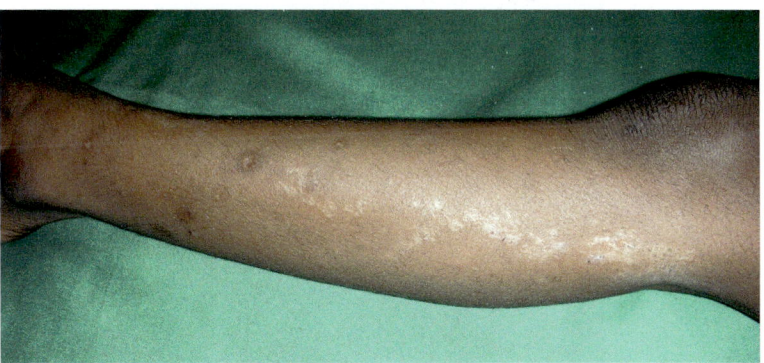

Figure 1.6 Lichen striatus is a benign, self-resolving condition, most typically seen in children. Elevated skin-colored papules coalesce to form one or more slightly scaly, hypopigmented, linear bands along Blaschko's lines.

Trauma. Intralesional steroids, post-thermal burns, post-dermatitis artefacta.

Other. Pigmentary demarcation lines, stretch marks, linear basaloid hamartoma.

1.7 Palmar pigmentation refers to the darkening or discoloration of palms caused by a variety of factors, including underlying medical conditions.[12]

Physiological. Pregnancy, Fitzpatrick skin type V and VI.

Inflammatory. Lichen planus, discoid lupus erythematosus, post-inflammatory hyperpigmentation (PIH).

Infections. Secondary syphilis, tinea nigra.

Metabolic. Carotenemia, pernicious anemia, vitamin B12 deficiency.

Endocrine. Addison's disease (Figure 1.7), Cushing's disease, carcinoid tumors and disease, pheochromocytoma, hypothyroidism, hyperthyroidism.

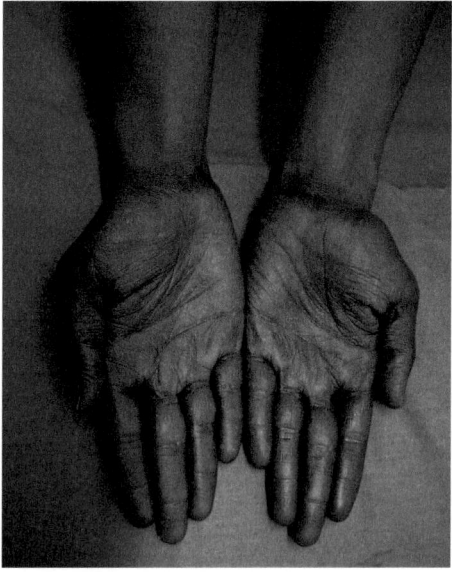

Figure 1.7 In Addison's disease, hyperpigmentation is caused by an excess of adrenocorticotropic hormone. It is usually generalized but is more evident in palmar creases.

Neoplasms. Acral melanoma, Bowen's disease, acanthosis nigricans secondary to malignancy.

Genetic. Alkaptonuria, reticulate acropigmentation of Kitamura, neurofibromatosis, Laugier–Hunziker syndrome, Cronkhite–Canada syndrome, Dowling–Degos disease, LEOPARD syndrome, POEMS syndrome, inherited patterned lentiginosis, Navajo neurohepatopathy.

Drug-related. Zidovudine, hydroxychloroquine, amiodarone, tetracyclines, 5-fluorouracil, hydroxyurea.

Other. Junctional nevus, arsenic poisoning, B12 deficiency, brown palm pseudochromhidrosis (use of tanning), PUVA therapy (psoralen plus ultraviolet A phototherapy), henna, post-potassium permanganate, exposure to silver (argyria)/gold/bismuth, trauma, amyloidosis, acromelanosis albo-punctata.

1.8 Reticulate acropigmentation is a net-like pattern of hyper- or hypopigmentation distributed along the distal extremities. Some of the causes are heritable, often with unique phenotypic characteristics.[13]

Inflammatory. Macular amyloidosis, scleroderma, phytophotodermatitis, PIH, erythema ab igne (Figure 1.8a).

Genetic. Reticulate acropigmentation of Kitamura, reticulate acropigmentation of Dohi, Haber's syndrome, Galli-Galli disease, epidermolysis bullosa, dermatopathia pigmentosa reticularis (Naegeli–

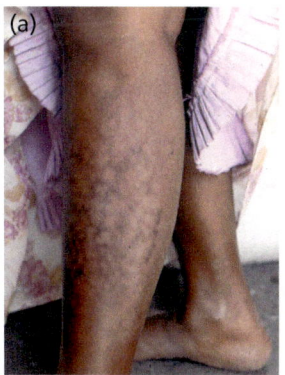
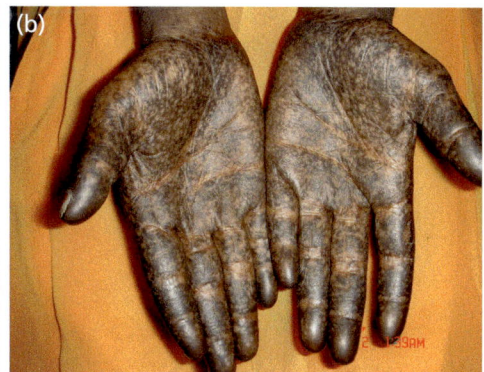

Figure 1.8 Reticulate acropigmentation caused by (a) erythema ab igne and (b) reaction to bleomycin.

Franceschetti–Jadassohn syndrome [mostly truncal]), Mendes da Costa–van der Valk syndrome, Hoyeraal–Hreidarsson syndrome, dyschromatosis universalis hereditaria, acromelanosis progressiva, incontinentia pigmenti.

Drug-related. Bleomycin (Figure 1.8b), diltiazem.

1.9 Oral pigmentation is a common manifestation in SOC. It can take the form of blue/purple vascular lesions, brown melanotic lesions, brown heme-associated lesions, or gray/black pigmentations.[14]

Physiological. Racial pigmentation, pregnancy, smoker's melanosis, melanocytic nevi.

Inflammatory. Oral lichen planus, post-immunobullous disorders.

Endocrine. Addison's disease.

Neoplasms. Malignant melanoma, Kaposi's sarcoma (Figure 1.9), oral melanoacanthoma.

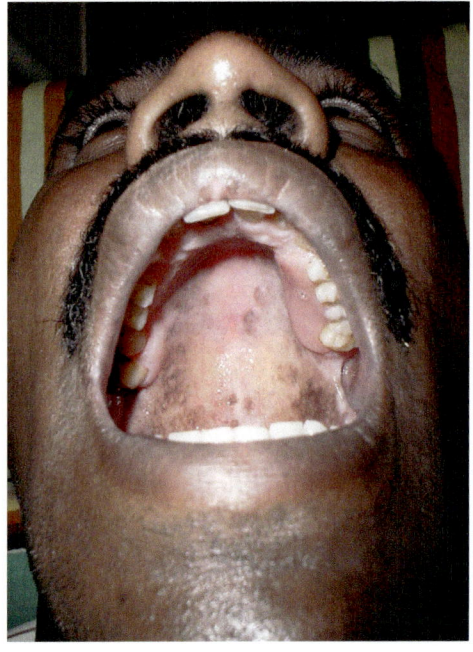

Figure 1.9 Kaposi's sarcoma in a patient with HIV infection.

Genetic. Peutz–Jeghers syndrome, Laugier–Hunziker syndrome, hemochromatosis.

Other. Oral melanotic macules, argyria, drug-induced (minocycline), lead and bismuth poisoning, amalgam tattoo, hairy tongue.

1.10 Pigmented tumors can be benign or malignant.[15] While a presumptive diagnosis can often be made by considering the history of the lesion and its location, appearance, and texture, along with the patient's risk factors, a definitive diagnosis must be made by biopsy and histological evaluation.

Benign. Seborrheic keratoses, skin tags (acrochordons), melanocytic nevi, dermatofibroma, syringoma, Bowenoid papulosis, angiokeratoma, neurofibroma (Figure 1.10a), hemangioma, lymphomatoid papulosis, pilomatricoma, mastocytoma, melanoacanthoma, trichoepithelioma (Figure 1.10b).

Malignant. Basal cell carcinoma, Bowen's disease, malignant melanoma, mycosis fungoides (cutaneous T-cell lymphoma; CTCL), Kaposi's sarcoma, Merkel cell carcinoma, Paget's disease.

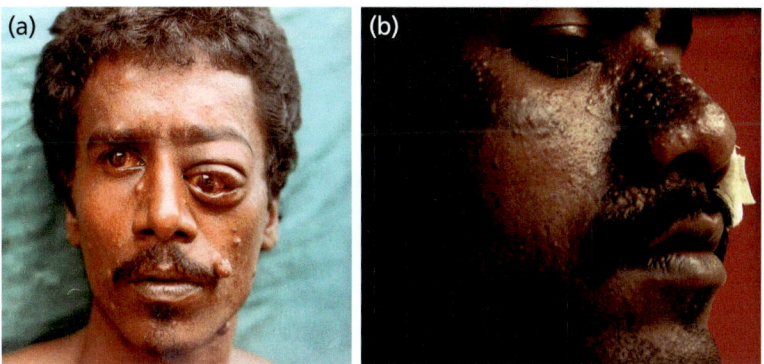

Figure 1.10 (a) Multiple cutaneous neurofibromas presenting as soft nodules on or under the skin. The patient also has a retro-orbital tumor causing eye displacement. (b) Multiple trichoepitheliomas arising from hair follicles. Trichoepitheliomas are mostly seen on the scalp, nose, forehead, and upper lip.

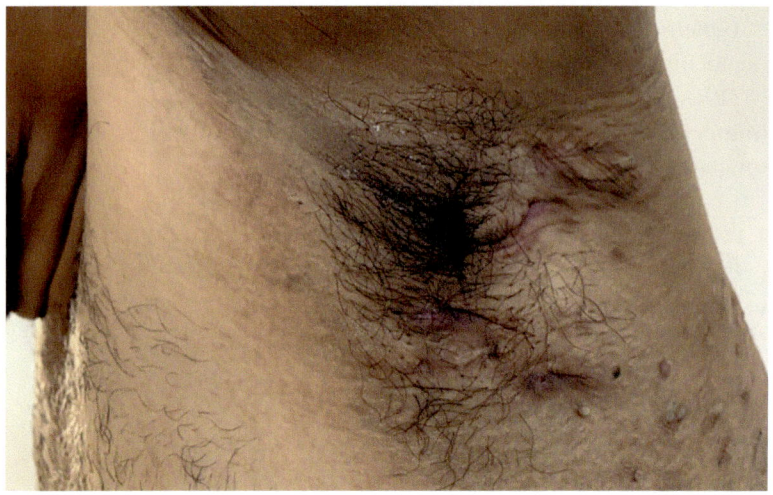

Figure 1.11 Hidradenitis suppurativa. Erythematous papules and bridged scars with comedones in the axilla.

Bumps, blisters, and pustules

1.11 Comedones are papules arising from follicular opening hyperkeratinization, giving the skin a bumpy appearance.[16]

Inflammatory. Acne (including infantile acne), hidradenitis suppurativa (HS) (Figure 1.11), chloracne, drug-induced acne, facial Afro-Caribbean childhood eruption.

Congenital. Comedo nevus.

Neoplasms. Mycosis fungoides.

Other. Radiation, pseudoacne of the transverse nasal crease, childhood flexural comedones, senile comedones of Favre–Racouchot syndrome, familial comedones, giant comedone.

1.12 Warty/verrucous dermatoses. There are various conditions that present with warty skin changes.[17]

Inflammatory. Lichen planus, sarcoidosis, psoriasis, verrucous lupus, keratosis lichenoides chronica, pemphigus vegetans.

Infections. Viral warts (human papillomavirus), tuberculosis verrucosa cutis, sporotrichosis, atypical mycobacteria, syphilis, verrucous lepromatous leprosy, chromoblastomycosis (Figure 1.12), crusted scabies, leishmaniasis, blastomycosis, dermatophytosis, herpes vegetans.

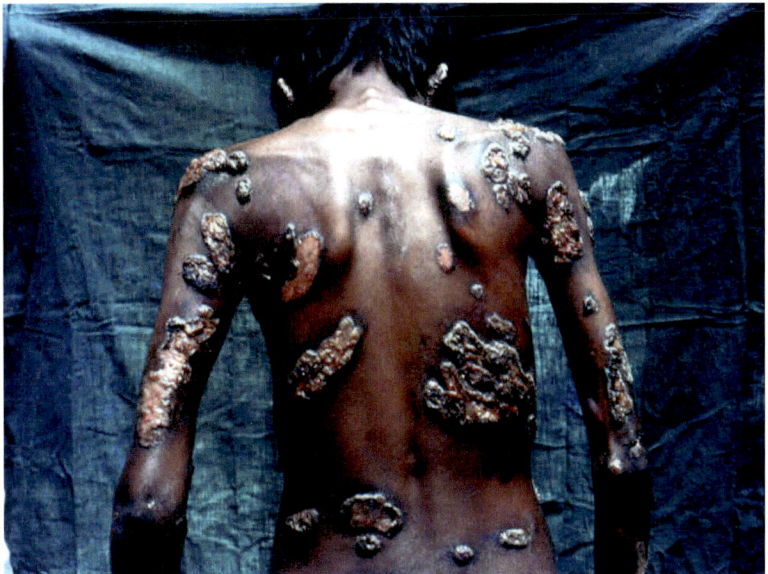

Figure 1.12 Chromoblastomycosis is a chronic granulomatous fungal infection that affects the skin and subcutaneous tissue. It presents as raised crusted lesions.

Congenital. Inflammatory linear verrucous epidermal nevus, Darier's disease, acrokeratosis verruciformis, verrucous porokeratosis, verrucous hemangioma, sebaceous nevus, incontinentia pigmenti.

Neoplasms. Mycosis fungoides, verrucous carcinoma (squamous cell carcinoma), verrucous melanoma, malignant acanthosis nigricans, verrucous Spitz nevus.

Other. Dermatosis neglecta, lymphedema.

1.13 Infantile blisters. Transient benign vesicles and bullae (small and large blisters containing clear fluid) in infants need to be differentiated from rare but life-threatening blistering diseases.[18]

Inflammatory. Chronic bullous dermatosis of childhood, bullous pemphigoid, eosinophilic pustular folliculitis, bullous lupus, maternal autoimmune bullous disease, pyoderma gangrenosum, bullous drug reaction.

Infections. Bullous impetigo (Figure 1.13), herpes simplex infection, herpes zoster infection, staphylococcal scalded-skin syndrome, varicella infection, scabies, congenital syphilis, intrauterine herpes simplex virus, congenital candidiasis, *Listeria monocytogenes,* cytomegalovirus (CMV), enterovirus, coxsackie virus, *Streptococcus, Malassezia* infection.

Neoplasms. Mastocytosis, Langerhans cell histiocytosis.

Metabolic. Acrodermatitis enteropathica.

Genetic. Epidermolysis bullosa, bullous congenital ichthyosiform erythroderma, porphyria, incontinentia pigmenti, Kindler's syndrome, ectodermal dysplasia (skin fragility), hyper-immunoglobulin (Ig) E syndrome, neonatal purpura fulminans.

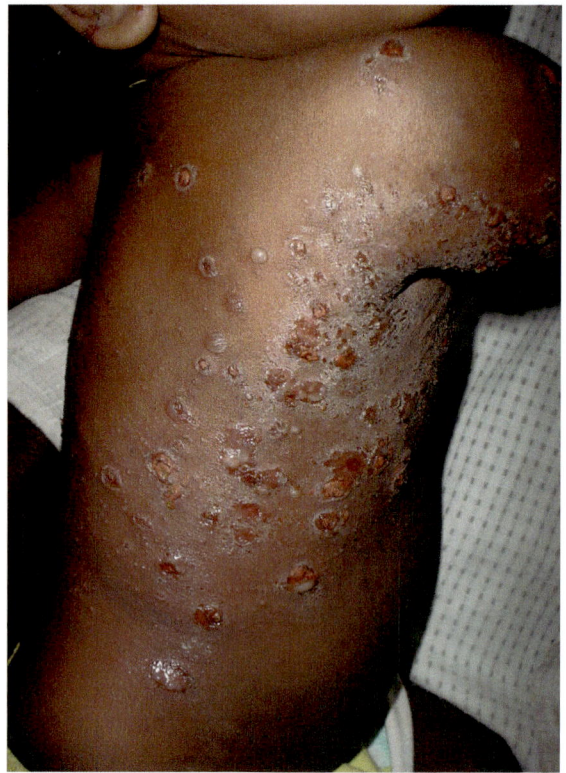

Figure 1.13 Bullous impetigo presents as fluid-filled blisters (bullae). It is caused by bacterial infections, almost exclusively *Staphylococcus aureus.*

Trauma. Sucking blisters, iatrogenic injury.

Other. Aplasia cutis, miliaria, intrauterine epidermal necrosis, hydroa vacciniforme, transient neonatal pustular melanosis, neonatal cephalic pustulosis, acropustulosis of infancy, erythema toxicum neonatorum.

1.14 Sterile pustules. Pustules are small blisters filled with inflammatory cells, predominantly neutrophils. Sterile pustules form in the absence of an infectious exudate.[19]

Inflammatory. Pustular psoriasis (Figure 1.14), irritant folliculitis, acropustulosis (may follow scabies infection), hyper-IgE syndrome, Behçet's disease.

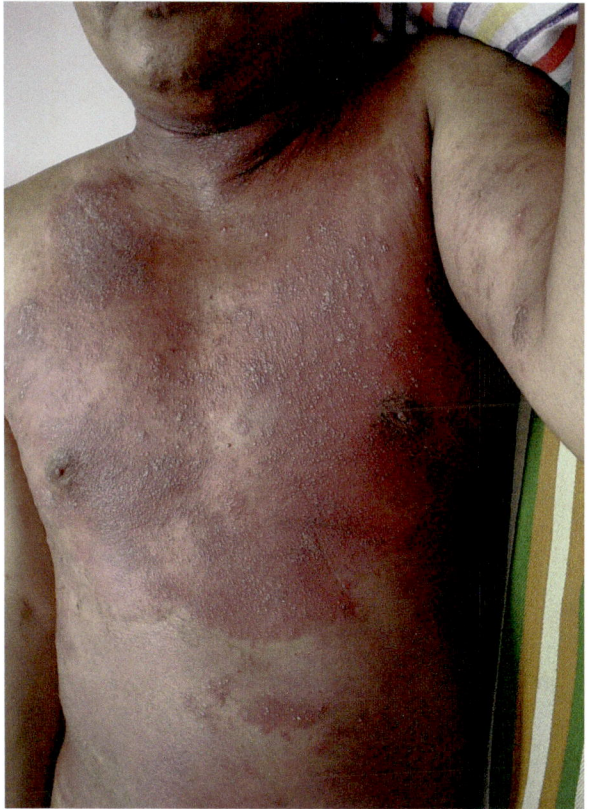

Figure 1.14 Pustular psoriasis.

Infections. *Pseudomonas*, post-viral infection, fungal id reaction.

Genetic. Incontinentia pigmenti, transient myeloproliferative disease in Down syndrome.

Other. Sucking blisters on fingers, miliaria.

1.15 Palmoplantar pustules are pus-filled blisters on the palms and soles. Identifying the underlying etiology is important as they can be difficult to treat.[20,21]

Inflammatory. Palmoplantar pustular psoriasis, pompholyx eczema, allergic contact dermatitis with secondary infection, acropustulosis of infancy, Behçet's disease, SAPHO syndrome, neonatal pustular melanosis, acrodermatitis continua of Hallopeau, acute graft-versus-host disease, Sweet's syndrome, subcorneal pustular dermatosis, Reiter's syndrome (reactive arthritis), pyoderma gangrenosum, pustular vasculitis, eosinophilic folliculitis.

Infections. Scabies, hand, foot, and mouth disease, tinea infection, impetigo, candidiasis, post-viral infection (Figure 1.15).

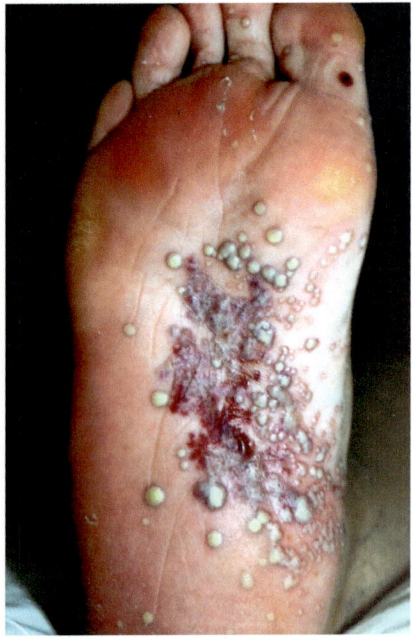

Figure 1.15 Post-viral pustular eruption on the sole of the foot.

Drug-related. Biologics-induced pustular psoriasis, acute generalized exanthematous pustulosis (AGEP), halogenoderma.

Lesions with a characteristic shape

1.16 Umbilicated lesions have a central depression or dimple.[22]

Inflammatory. Lichen planus, prurigo nodularis, hydroa vacciniforme, sarcoidosis, granuloma annulare, palisaded neutrophilic granulomatous dermatitis.

Infections. Molluscum contagiosum, eczema herpeticum, herpes zoster, cryptococcosis, histoplasmosis, coccidioidomycosis, mpox (Figure 1.16), smallpox, leprosy, viral warts, cowpox, orf, milker's nodule, talaromycosis (formerly penicilliosis), sporotrichosis.

Neoplasms. Basal cell carcinoma, keratoacanthoma, porocarcinoma, leukemia cutis.

Benign lesions. Trichofolliculoma, fibrous adenoma, desmoplastic trichoepithelioma, juvenile xanthogranuloma, epidermoid cyst, Spitz nevus, sebaceous hyperplasia, warty dyskeratoma.

Other. Pityriasis rosea (vesicular type), eruptive xanthoma, perforating disorders, Degos disease, folliculitis, acrokeratoelastoidosis of Costa.

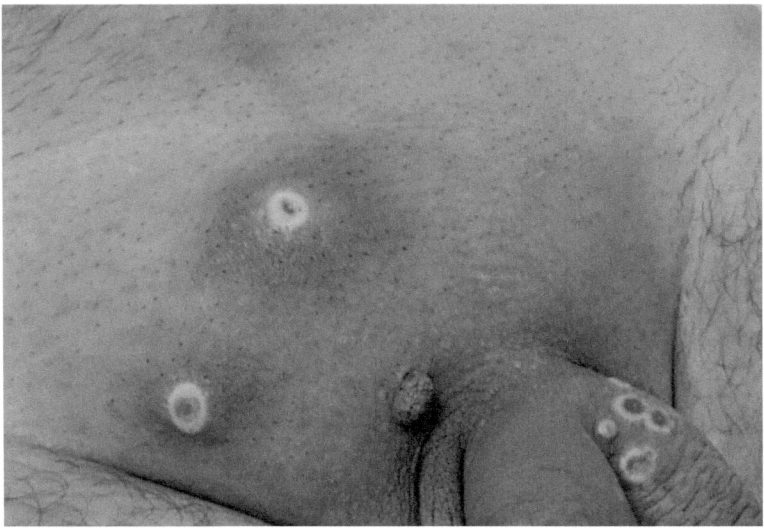

Figure 1.16 Umbilicated vesicles and pustules of mpox.

1.17 Serpiginous lesions have a winding and curved shape, resembling a snake.[23]

Inflammatory. Lichen striatus, subacute cutaneous lupus erythematosus, erythema annulare centrifugum, granuloma annulare, linear IgA bullous dermatosis, subcorneal pustular dermatosis, urticaria, purpura annularis telangiectodes of Majocchi (Majocchi's disease), erythema multiforme, sarcoidosis, pemphigus foliaceus, seborrheic eczema, annular erythema of infancy, erythema dyschromicum perstans, balanitis circinata, eosinophilic annular erythema, jellyfish sting.

Infections. Larva migrans (Figure 1.17), scabies, tinea corporis, erythema chronicum migrans, tertiary syphilis.

Neoplasms. Erythema gyratum repens, mycosis fungoides, necrolytic migratory erythema.

Genetic. Epidermal nevus, porokeratosis, incontinentia pigmenti (third stage), hypomelanosis of Ito, erythrokeratodermia variabilis, ichthyosis hystrix.

Other. Elastosis perforans serpiginosa, arthropod infection, angioma serpiginosum.

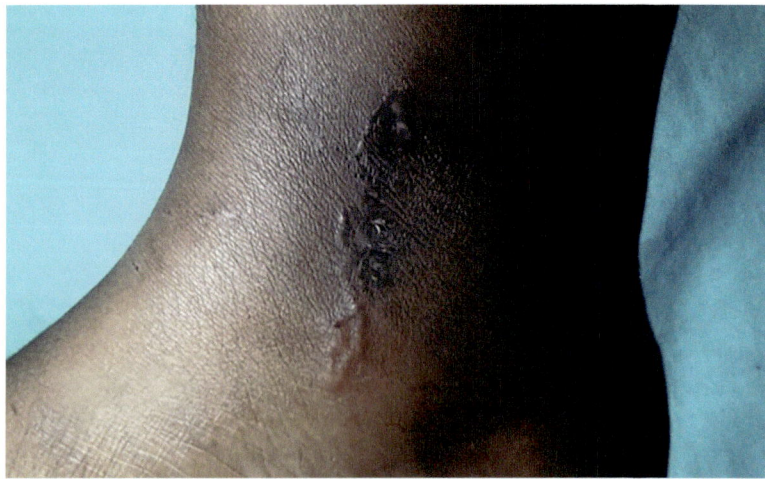

Figure 1.17 Cutaneous larva migrans, a parasitic skin infection caused by hookworm larvae, manifests as an erythematous, serpiginous, pruritic cutaneous eruption.

1.18 Annular lesions are ring-shaped with a raised border.[24]

Inflammatory. Erythema annulare centrifugum, erythema multiforme, granuloma annulare, pityriasis rosea, discoid lupus erythematosus, subacute cutaneous lupus erythematosus, sarcoidosis, alopecia mucinosa, Jessner's lymphocytic infiltrate, polymorphous light eruption, neonatal lupus erythematosus, Sweet's syndrome, parapsoriasis, fixed drug eruption, psoriasis (Figure 1.18), annular lichen planus, subcorneal pustular dermatosis, urticaria, insect bite reaction, seborrheic dermatitis, urticarial vasculitis, necrobiosis lipoidica, linear IgA bullous dermatosis, granuloma multiforme, morphea, erythema marginatum, annular lichenoid dermatitis of youth, familial annular erythema, IgA vasculitis, hemorrhagic edema of infancy, annular erythema of infancy, Wells' syndrome, purpura annularis telangiectodes of Majocchi, granuloma faciale.

Infections. Secondary and tertiary syphilis, tinea corporis, impetigo, cutaneous larva migrans, leishmaniasis, leprosy, lupus vulgaris, Lyme disease, tertiary yaws.

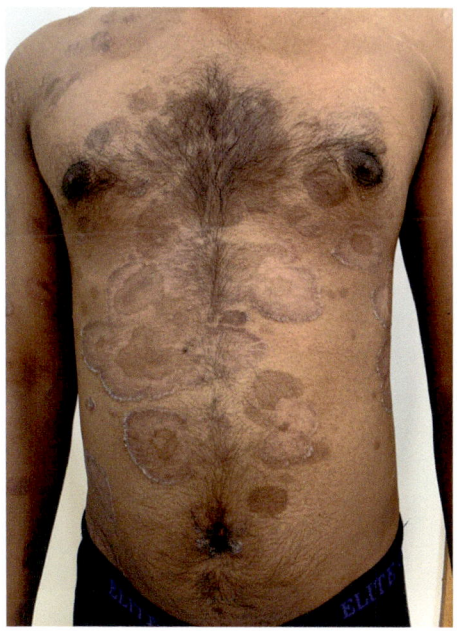

Figure 1.18 Resolving plaques of psoriasis showing an annular morphology.

Neoplasms/paraneoplastic conditions. CTCL, leukemia/lymphoma cutis, erythema gyratum repens.

Other. Ichthyosis linearis circumflexa, porokeratosis, elastosis perforans serpiginosa, actinic granuloma, Meyerson's nevus, erythrokeratodermia, cupping, dermatitis artefacta.

Dermatoses with a specific pattern or distribution

1.19 Migratory dermatoses. A migratory rash appears in one area of the body before spreading to other parts, often in a wave-like pattern.[25]

Classic migratory rashes. Erythema annulare centrifugum, erythema gyratum repens, erythema marginatum, erythema chronicum migrans.

Creeping eruptions. Cutaneous larva migrans (Figure 1.19), dirofilariasis, fascioliasis, gnathostomiasis, loiasis.

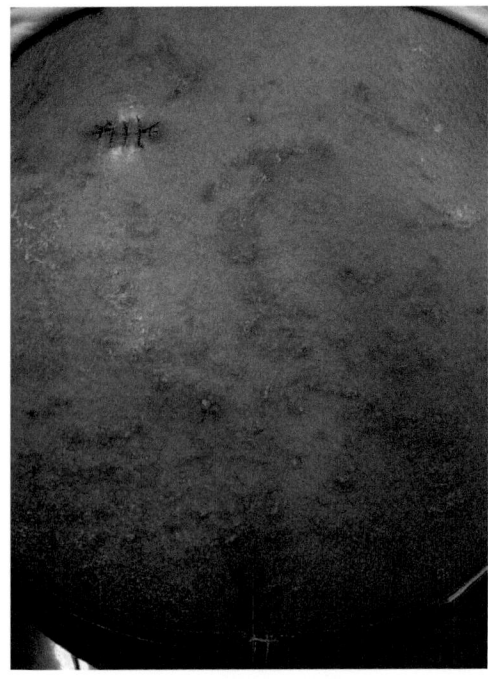

Figure 1.19 A creeping eruption caused by florid cutaneous larva migrans infestation.

Other. Urticaria, tinea, erythrokeratodermia variabilis, necrolytic migratory erythema.

1.20 Linear morphology is common. It may result from lesions following Blaschko's lines, blood vessels, lymphatic vessels, or dermatomes.[26,27]

Physiological. Futcher's lines, linea nigra, striae atrophicans, linea alba.

Inflammatory. Psoriasis, lichen nitidus, chronic graft-versus-host disease, lichen planus (Figure 1.20a), lichen striatus, morphea (en coup de sabre) (Figure 1.20b), lupus erythematosus, pemphigus, segmental vitiligo, fixed-drug eruption, linear atrophoderma of Moulin, *Paederus* dermatitis (Figure 1.20c), berloque dermatitis, pityriasis rosea, all causes of blaschkitis.

Infections. Verruca, molluscum contagiosum, herpes zoster, larva migrans, scabetic burrows, lymphangitis, sporotrichosis.

Genetic. Goltz syndrome, incontinentia pigmenti, Hailey–Hailey disease, inflammatory linear verrucous epidermal nevus, Darier's disease, hypomelanosis of Ito, linear and whorled nevoid

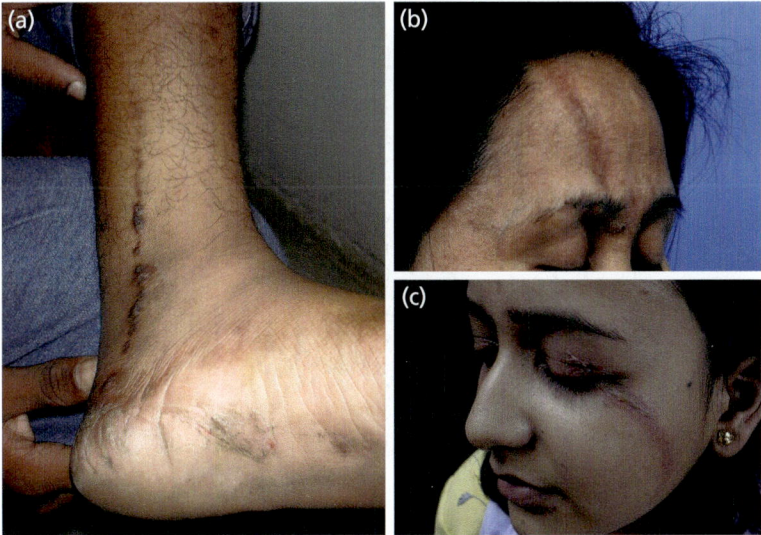

Figure 1.20 (a) Linear lesions of lichen planus on the lower leg. (b) Linear morphea (en coup de sabre). (c) *Paederus* dermatitis, a linear erythema caused by paederin, a fluid released by a beetle from the *Paederus* genus.

hypermelanosis, bullous ichthyosiform erythroderma, epidermal nevi, linear Cowden's nevus, porokeratosis, nevus depigmentosus, nevus lipomatosus superficialis.

Neoplasms. Basal cell carcinoma, eccrine spiradenoma, basaloid follicular hamartoma, connective tissue nevus, segmental angiofibroma, syringoma, segmental leiomyoma, zosteriform lentiginous nevus, trichoepithelioma, segmental neurofibroma.

Trauma/external. Dermatitis artefacta, insect bites and stings, phytophotodermatitis, phytodermatitis.

Other. Unilateral nevoid telangiectasia, fibromatosis, thrombophlebitis, nevus corniculatus, linear focal elastosis, nevus comedonicus, nevus sebaceous, porokeratotic eccrine ostial and dermal duct nevus, palmoplantar verrucous nevus, flagellate conditions.

1.21 Digitate dermatoses are characterized by elongated finger-like projections or branches (Figure 1.21).[28,29]

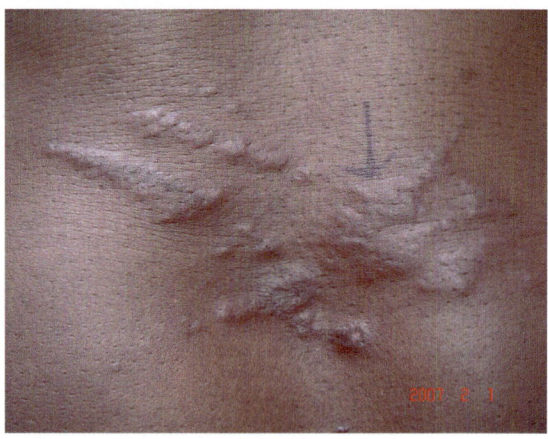

Figure 1.21 Digitate dermatosis caused by bleomycin toxicity.

Inflammatory. Contact dermatitis, lichen planus, lupus erythematosus, nummular eczema, pityriasis alba, pityriasis rosea, pityriasis lichenoides chronica, psoriasis.

Infections. Secondary syphilis, leprosy.

Neoplasms. Mycosis fungoides, lymphomatoid papulosis.

Other. Pityriasis rosea-like drug eruption bleomycin toxicity (see Figure 1.21).

1.22 Christmas-tree pattern. Also called pityriasis rosea-like eruption (Figure 1.22), Christmas tree rashes are distributed on the trunk like a Christmas tree or along skin creases.[30,31]

Inflammatory. Pityriasis lichenoides, disseminated contact dermatitis, nummular eczema, lichen planus, erythema dyschromicum perstans, seborrheic dermatitis, Gianotti–Crosti syndrome, small

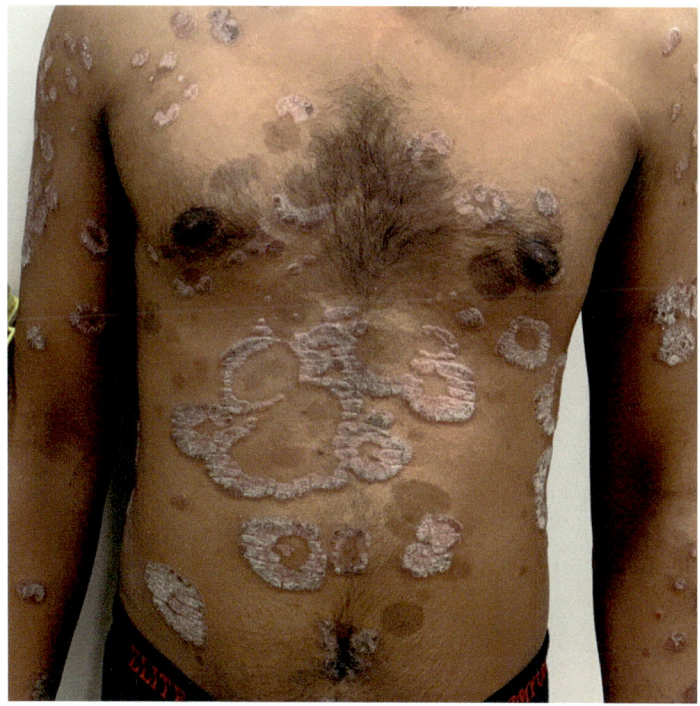

Figure 1.22 Pityriasis rosea-like eruption.

plaque parapsoriasis, erythema annulare centrifugum, guttate psoriasis, erythema multiforme, lupus erythematosus purpura, dermatophyte id reaction.

Infections. Viral exanthems, secondary syphilis, HIV exanthem, tinea versicolor, tinea corporis, scabies, COVID-19.

Neoplasms. Kaposi's sarcoma (HIV associated), mycosis fungoides, leukemia (deposits).

Drug-related (pityriasis rosea-like drug reaction). ACE inhibitors, omeprazole, clonidine, isotretinoin, metronidazole, barbiturates, gold, beta-blockers, D-penicillamine, griseofulvin, imatinib mesylate, ondansetron, COVID-19 vaccination.

1.23 Sporotrichoid distribution. Sporotrichoid morphology takes the appearance of subcutaneous nodules distributed along lymphatic vessels.[32]

Inflammatory. Sarcoidosis.

Infections. Sporotrichosis (Figure 1.23), atypical mycobacteria, leishmaniasis, tuberculosis, cat scratch disease, pyogenic diseases,

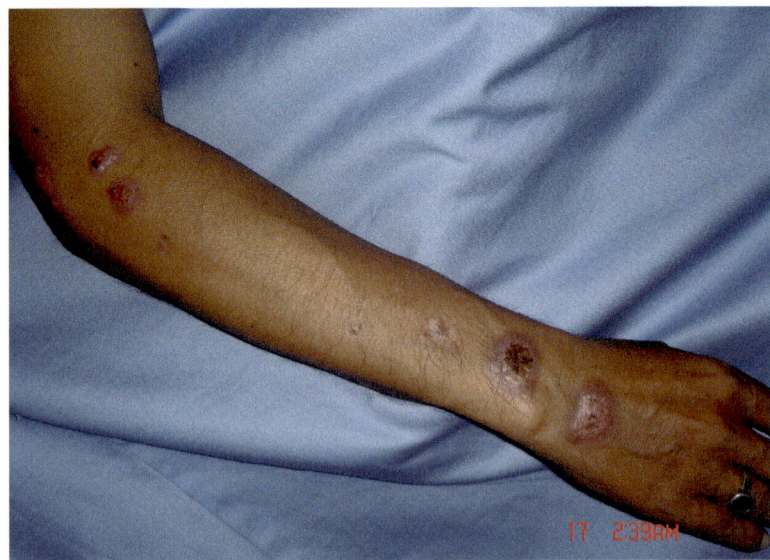

Figure 1.23 Sporotrichosis, a fungal infection caused by *Sporothrix schenckii*, showing nodules along the lymphatic vessels.

nocardiosis, mycetoma, chromoblastomycosis, anthrax, coccidioidomycosis, syphilis, lepromatous leprosy, cowpox, pasteurella, tularemia, multiple nerve abscesses, intravenous drug addicts (bacterial infections).
Neoplasms. Metastatic deposits, mycosis fungoides.

1.24 Zosteriform/blaschkoid dermatoses are restricted to dermatomal distribution or along the lines of Blaschko, which represent embryonic growth patterns during epidermal cell migration.[33]

Inflammatory. Lichen planus, vitiligo, lichen striatus, lichen sclerosus, pityriasis lichenoides, contact dermatitis (including phytophotodermatitis), morphea, granuloma annulare, bullous pemphigoid, graft-versus-host disease, photoallergic reaction, pemphigus, lichen aureus, caterpillar dermatitis, blaschkitis.

Infections. Herpes zoster, zosteriform herpes simplex, bullous impetigo, candidiasis, infectious folliculitis, erysipelas, cellulitis.

Genetic. Incontinentia pigmenti, Darier's disease, neurofibromatosis, X-linked chondrodysplasia punctata.

Neoplasms. Zosteriform secondary cutaneous metastasis, cutaneous T- and B-cell lymphomas, squamous cell carcinoma, Kaposi's sarcoma, angiosarcoma, melanocytic and connective tissue hamartomas, trichoepitheliomas.

Other. Becker's nevus, epidermal nevus (Figure 1.24), progressive cribriform and zosteriform hyperpigmentation, perforating collagenosis, linear atrophoderma of Moulin, porokeratosis, hypomelanosis of Ito, nevus of Ota.

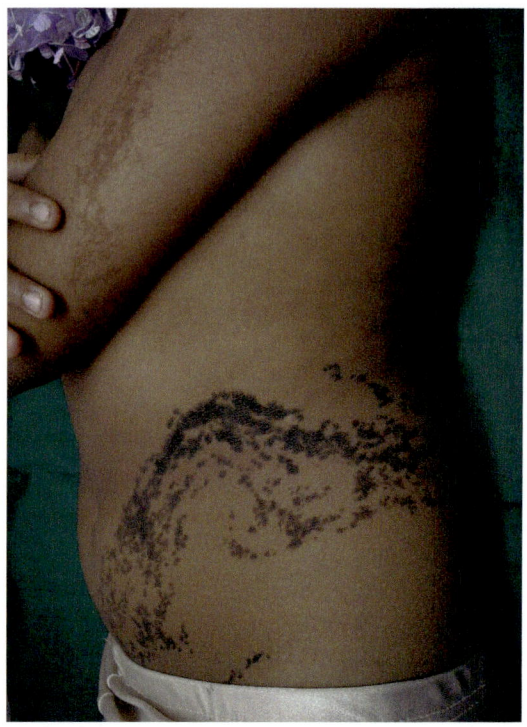

Figure 1.24 Epidermal nevus along the lines of Blaschko.

Pathergy

1.25 Pathergy refers to the hyper-reaction of the skin to minor trauma. It is most often seen in Behçet's disease but can occur in other dermatoses as well.[34,35]

Inflammatory. Behçet's disease, pyoderma gangrenosum (Figure 1.25), neutrophilic eccrine hidradenitis, erythema elevatum diutinum, systemic lupus erythematosus, Sweet's syndrome, eosinophilic pustular folliculitis, Crohn's disease, pemphigus foliaceus, pemphigoid, subcorneal pustular dermatosis, PAPA syndrome.

Neoplasms. Chronic myeloid leukemia (myeloproliferative disorders).

Genetic. Neonates with Down syndrome.

Other. Calciphylaxis, blind loop syndrome, healthy individuals.

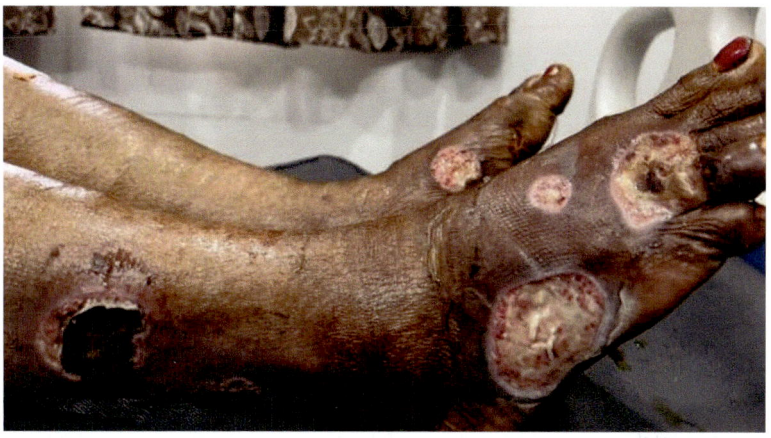

Figure 1.25 Pyoderma gangrenosum, showing ulcers with a violaceous margin.

Perforating disorders

1.26a Primary perforating disorders are a group of conditions characterized by abnormal keratinization and transepidermal elimination. The four primary perforating dermatoses are elastosis perforans serpiginosa, reactive perforating collagenosis, perforating folliculitis, and Kyrle's disease (Figure 1.26).[36]

Other conditions that exhibit transepidermal elimination include:

Inflammatory. Lichen nitidus, granulomatous conditions (granuloma annulare, necrobiosis lipoidica, rheumatoid nodule, sarcoid), hidradenitis, chondrodermatitis nodularis, vitiligo.

Infiltrative. Amyloidosis, papular mucinosis.

Infections. Tuberculosis, leishmaniasis, chromoblastomycosis, lobomycosis, botryomycosis, schistosomiasis, histoid leprosy, rhinosporidiosis.

Neoplasms. Melanoma, eruptive vellus hair cysts.

Genetic. Pseudoxanthoma elasticum, focal dermal hypoplasia.

Other. Porokeratosis, gout, tattoo pigment, foreign body, calcinosis cutis, osteoma cutis, perforating calcific elastosis.

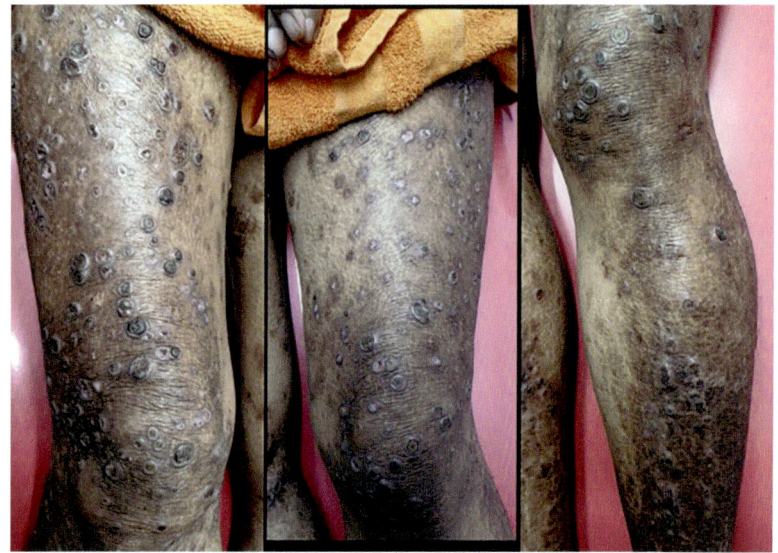

Figure 1.26 Kyrle's disease, showing keratotic papules and nodules in both lower limbs in a patient with diabetes.

1.26b Secondary (acquired) perforating disorders are due to kidney failure or diabetes.[37]

Skin conditions masquerading as common dermatoses

1.27 Lichenoid dermatoses are characterized by lichen planus-like morphology. They usually present as flat-topped, shiny, purple, papular eruptions.[38]

Inflammatory. Lichen planus, lichen nitidus (Figure 1.27a), lichenoid contact dermatitis, lichenoid pigmented purpuric dermatosis, lichen striatus, lichen scrofulosorum, pityriasis lichenoides, pityriasis lichenoides et varioliformis acuta (PLEVA), lichenoid sarcoidosis, lichen simplex, lichenoid graft-versus-host disease, lichen spinulosus, keratosis lichenoides chronica, lichen myxedematosus, lichen amyloidosis, lichen aureus, annular lichenoid dermatitis of youth.

Infections. Lichenoid secondary syphilis, Gianotti–Crosti syndrome.

Neoplasms and benign lesions. Lichenoid mycosis fungoides, lichenoid keratosis, lichenoid actinic keratosis, disseminated superficial actinic porokeratosis (DSAP).

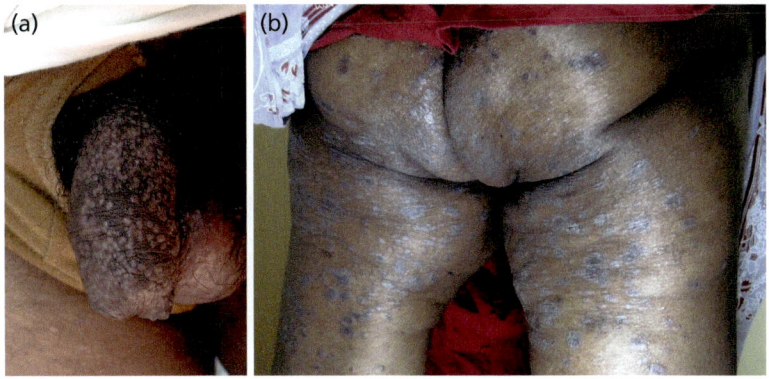

Figure 1.27 (a) Lichen nitidus. (b) Lichenoid eruption caused by imatinib.

Other. Lichenoid drug eruption (Figure 1.27b), frictional lichenoid dermatosis.

1.28 Psoriasiform dermatoses. This group is characterized by psoriasiform morphology that mimics psoriasis clinically.[39]

Inflammatory. Psoriasis vulgaris (Figure 1.28), contact dermatitis (irritant/allergic), seborrheic eczema, pityriasis rosea, atopic eczema/nummular eczema, lichen simplex, pityriasis rubra pilaris, chronic prurigo, lichen planus, pityriasis lichenoides, sarcoidosis, subacute cutaneous lupus, dermatomyositis, systemic lupus, reactive arthritis syndrome, chronic actinic dermatitis, graft-versus-host disease, capillaritis (pigmented purpura), pemphigus foliaceus, pompholyx eczema.

Infections. Syphilis, tinea corporis, Norwegian scabies, chronic candidiasis, viral eruptions, tuberculosis verrucosa cutis, erythema chronicum migrans, COVID-19 related, chromoblastomycosis, pityriasis versicolor.

Neoplasms. Mycosis fungoides, Bowen's disease, glucagonoma, Bazex syndrome, Hodgkin's lymphoma.

Metabolic. Pellagra, acrodermatitis enteropathica, acquired zinc deficiency.

Genetic. Inflammatory linear verrucous epidermal nevus, lamellar ichthyosis, erythrokeratoderma variabilis.

Other. Drug eruptions.

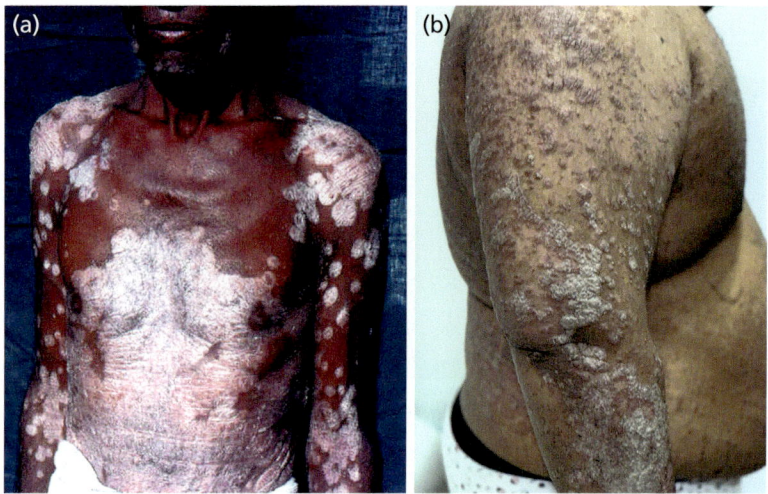

Figure 1.28 (a) Severe plaque psoriasis vulgaris. (b) Hyperkeratotic psoriasis.

1.29 Acneiform dermatoses can mimic classic acne.[40–42]

Inflammatory. Acne vulgaris (Figure 1.29a), perioral dermatitis, HS, occupational (chloracne), halogenoderma (iodides, bromides), chemical acne (heavy oils, waxes, cutting oils), pomade acne (hair oils), sarcoidosis, Fox–Fordyce disease, acne aestivalis, idiopathic facial aseptic granuloma, pseudofolliculitis barbae, eosinophilic pustular folliculitis.

Infections. Pityrosporum (Malassezia) folliculitis, Demodex folliculitis (Figure 1.29b), Gram-negative folliculitis (Proteus, Klebsiella, Escherichia coli, Enterobacter), syphilis, mycotic infection, hot tub folliculitis, tinea barbae, flat warts, molluscum contagiosum, herpes simplex, sporotrichosis, coccidioidomycosis.

Neoplasms. Mycosis fungoides.

Genetic. Nevus comedonicus, eruptive vellus hair cysts, tuberous sclerosis.

Drug-related. Corticosteroids, anabolic steroids, testosterone, lithium, ciclosporin, vitamin B12, anticonvulsants, macrolides, isoniazid, naproxen, hydroxychloroquine, epidermal growth factor receptor (EGFR) inhibitors, tumor necrosis factor (TNF)α inhibitors.

Other. Friction, pressure, post-radiation.

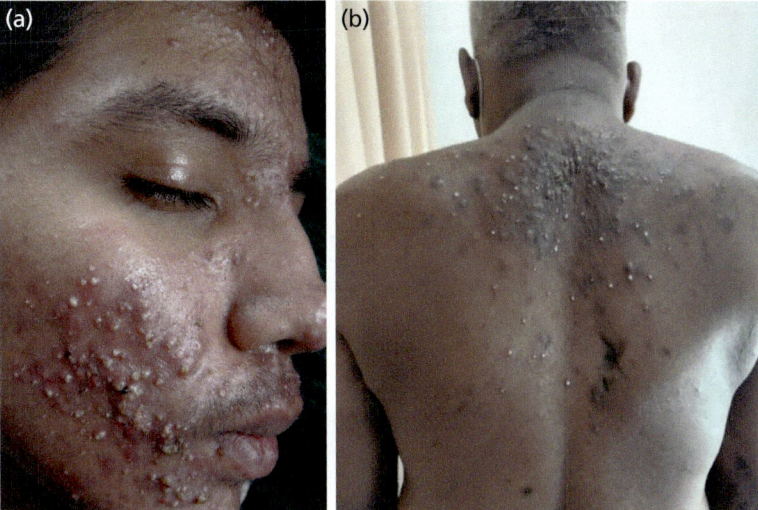

Figure 1.29 (a) Acne vulgaris. (b) *Demodex* plus *Pityrosporum* (*Malassezia*) folliculitis in a patient after a kidney transplant.

1.30 Pellagra-like dermatoses (Figure 1.30). Pellagra is caused by a lack of niacin (vitamin B3) or its precursor tryptophan in the diet, making skin cells more photosensitive. It causes a distinctive dermatitis that initially looks like sunburn before progressing to rough, scaly, hyperpigmented plaques.[43,44]

Inflammatory. Lupus erythematosus, chronic actinic dermatitis, actinic reticuloid, seborrheic dermatitis, contact dermatitis, pemphigus erythematosus, polymorphous light eruption, granular parakeratosis, photosensitive drug reaction.

Infections. HIV infection.

Neoplasms. Carcinoid tumor.

Metabolic. Kwashiorkor, zinc deficiency, malabsorption syndrome, bariatric surgery, pyridoxine deficiency, B2/B6/B12 deficiency, excessive alcohol.

Genetic. Erythropoietic protoporphyria, variegate porphyria, Hartnup's syndrome, porphyria cutanea tarda.

Drug-related. Isoniazid, 5-fluorouracil, azathioprine, 6-mercaptopurine.

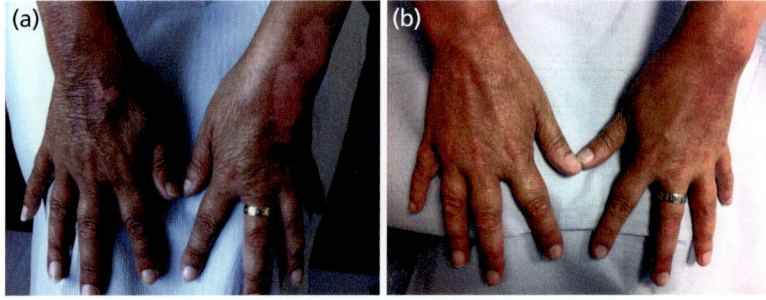

Figure 1.30 Pellagra (a) before and (b) after treatment.

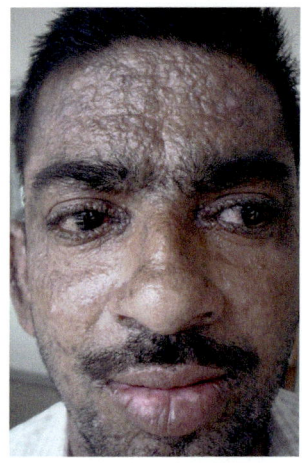

Figure 1.31 Varioliform scarring caused by lipoid proteinosis.

1.31 Varioliform scarring is characterized by sharply demarcated flesh-colored depressions (Figure 1.31), which resemble variola virus infection (smallpox).[45]

Inflammatory. Acne vulgaris, HS, hydroa vacciniforme, acne necrotica (necrotic lymphocytic folliculitis), PLEVA, papulonecrotic tuberculid, atrophoderma vermiculatum, actinic prurigo, pseudoporphyria, folliculitis decalvans, atrophia maculosa varioliformis cutis (AMVS), lupus miliaris disseminatus faciei.

Infections. Smallpox, varicella, echovirus, scarring from atypical mycobacterium.

Neoplasms. Lymphomatoid papulosis, hydroa-like cutaneous lymphoma.
Genetic. Erythropoietic protoporphyria, lipoid proteinosis (see Figure 1.31).
Other. Malignant atrophic papulosis.

1.32 Photosensitive disorders in children. Photosensitivity should be suspected if the child develops sunburn despite limited sun exposure. Early recognition ensures appropriate photoprotection, and an accurate diagnosis can help to minimize long-term complications.[46,47]
Inflammatory. Polymorphic light eruption (Figure 1.32), chronic actinic dermatitis, connective tissue diseases, psoriasis, photoaggravated eczema, seborrheic eczema, lupus, juvenile spring eruption, actinic prurigo, hydroa vacciniforme, solar urticaria.
Infections. Herpes simplex, herpes zoster.
Metabolic. Pellagra.

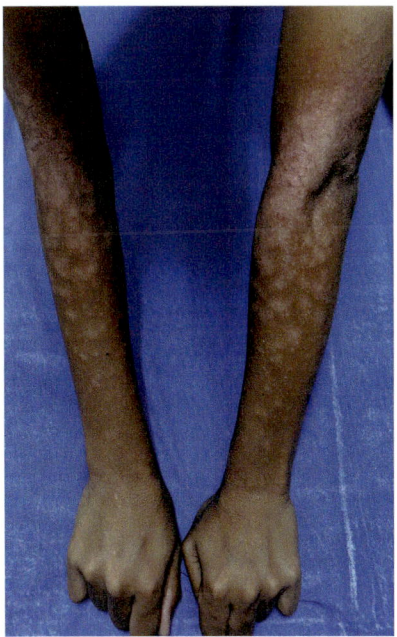

Figure 1.32 Polymorphic light eruption.

Genetic. Xeroderma pigmentosum, Cockayne syndrome, COFS syndrome, UV-sensitive syndrome, porphyria cutanea tarda, erythropoietic protoporphyria, phenylketonuria, trichothiodystrophy, Bloom syndrome, Rothmund–Thomson syndrome.

Chemical- and drug-related. Topical agents (photoallergic), herbal remedies (St John's wort), furanocoumarins (photosensitizing chemicals in plant sap and fruits, causing phytophotodermatitis).

Other. Sunburn.

Dermatoses of the face and ears

1.33 Leonine facies is characterized by facial features resembling a lion, with prominent folds of skin and furrows on the face and scalp.[48]

Inflammatory. Actinic reticuloid, scleromyxedema, sarcoidosis, granulomatous rosacea.

Infections. Lepromatous leprosy, PKDL (Figure 1.33), syphilis.

Endocrine. Hyperthyroidism, hypothyroidism, acromegaly.

Neoplasms. Mycosis fungoides (CTCL),[48] leukemia cutis, multicentric reticulohistiocytosis, Kaposi's sarcoma, carcinoid tumors and disease, sebaceous hyperplasia.

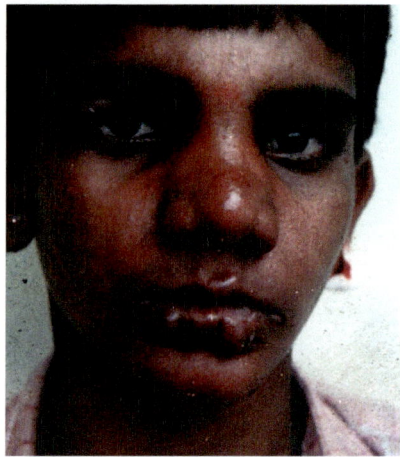

Figure 1.33 Swollen nose and lips of post-kala-azar dermal leishmaniasis (PKDL). PKDL is a progressive disease that can lead to a leonine facies appearance.

Genetic. Lipoid proteinosis, pachydermoperiostosis, phenylketonuria, Grzybowski's syndrome.
Other. Paget's disease, amyloidosis, mastocytosis.

1.34 Destructive nasal lesions. A variety of conditions can cause destruction of the skin, cartilage, and bone forming the nasal structure.
Inflammatory. Granulomatosis with polyangiitis, sarcoidosis, relapsing polychondritis, Goodpasture's syndrome, systemic lupus erythematosus, pyoderma gangrenosum, Ig G4-related disease, polyarteritis nodosa, Takayasu's arteritis, Behçet's disease.
Infections. Leprosy, lupus vulgaris, leishmaniasis, blastomycosis, bejel (endemic syphilis), actinomycosis, paracoccidioidomycosis, yaws (gangosa), mucormycosis, rhinosporidiosis, noma, tertiary syphilis, zygomycosis, rhinoscleroma, rhinoentomophthoromycosis.
Neoplasms. Basal cell carcinoma, squamous cell carcinoma, natural killer (NK) cell lymphoma (lethal midline granuloma), eosinophilic granuloma, sarcoma, rhabdomyosarcoma, lobular capillary hemangioma.
Other. Cocaine abuse, trigeminal trophic syndrome (Figure 1.34), intranasal steroid injection, chronic nose picking.

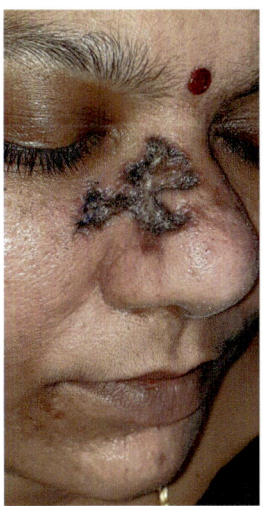

Figure 1.34 Trigeminal trophic syndrome is a rare cause of facial ulceration following damage to the trigeminal nerve or its central sensory pathways.

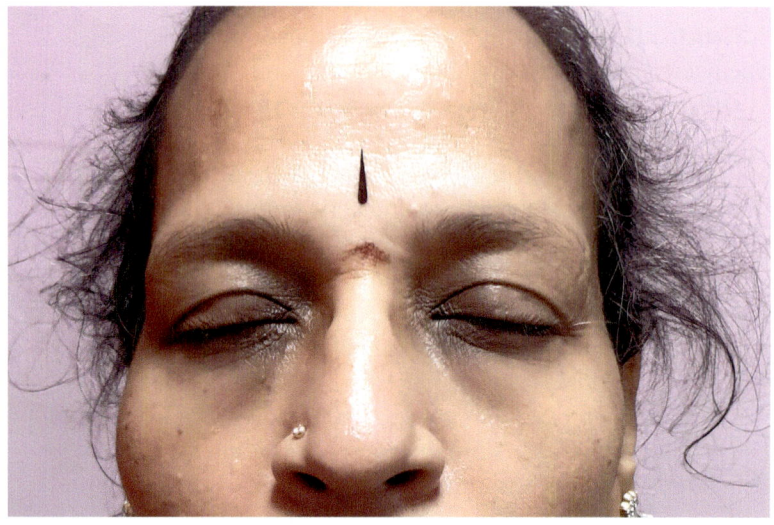

Figure 1.35 Loss of lateral one-third of eyebrow.

1.35 Loss of the lateral one-third of the eyebrows (Figure 1.35) is also called Hertoghe's or Queen Anne's sign. It can be caused by constant scratching and rubbing due to an inflammatory condition, or it is sometimes the presenting sign of a systemic condition.[49]

Inflammatory. Atopic eczema, alopecia areata, sarcoidosis, lichen planopilaris.

Infections. Lepromatous leprosy, syphilis.

Endocrine. Hypothyroidism, hypoparathyroidism.

Localized (tend to be unilateral). Post-infection, post-trauma, discoid lupus erythematosus, trichotillomania, Parry–Rhomberg syndrome (progressive facial hemiatrophy).

Other. Heavy metal poisoning, Dubowitz syndrome, follicular mucinosis, ulerythema ophryogenes, ectodermal dysplasia.

1.36 Thickened pinnae. Thickening of the external ear can sometimes be a manifestation of infections and serious systemic disorders.[50]

Inflammatory. Sarcoidosis, scleromyxedema, contact dermatitis, otophyma (rosacea), granuloma faciale, cutaneous Crohn's disease, granuloma annulare, chronic actinic dermatitis, chondrodermatitis nodularis helicis, lupus erythematosus.

Differential diagnoses by history and clinical features

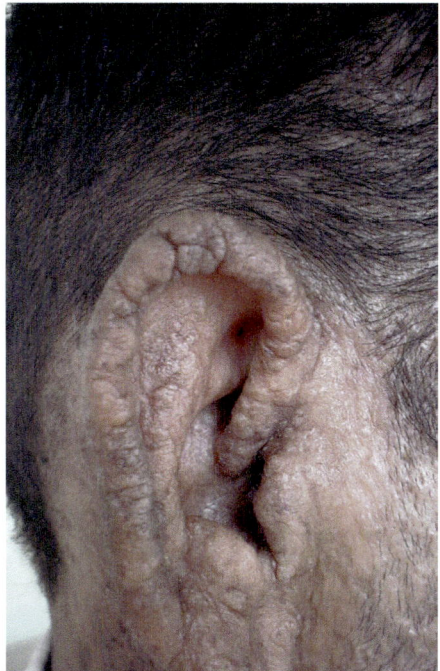

Figure 1.36 Lipoid proteinosis causing thickening of the pinnae.

Infections. Lepromatous leprosy, PKDL, lupus vulgaris.
Congenital. Lipoid proteinosis (Figure 1.36), mucopolysaccharidosis, juvenile hyaline fibromatosis.
Neoplasms. Mycosis fungoides, Bowen's disease, lymphocytoma, Waldenström's macroglobulinemia, IgG4 skin disease.
Other. Keloid, myxedema, acromegaly, amyloidosis, angiolymphoid hyperplasia with eosinophilia, hemangioma, pyogenic granuloma, milia en plaque, xanthomatosis.

Dermatoses of the nails and palms

1.37 Pseudo-Hutchinson sign. The presence of subungual pigmentation in the absence of features of subungual melanoma is termed the 'pseudo-Hutchinson' sign (Figure 1.37).[51]

Infections. Pseudomonas.
Neoplasms. Bowen's disease.

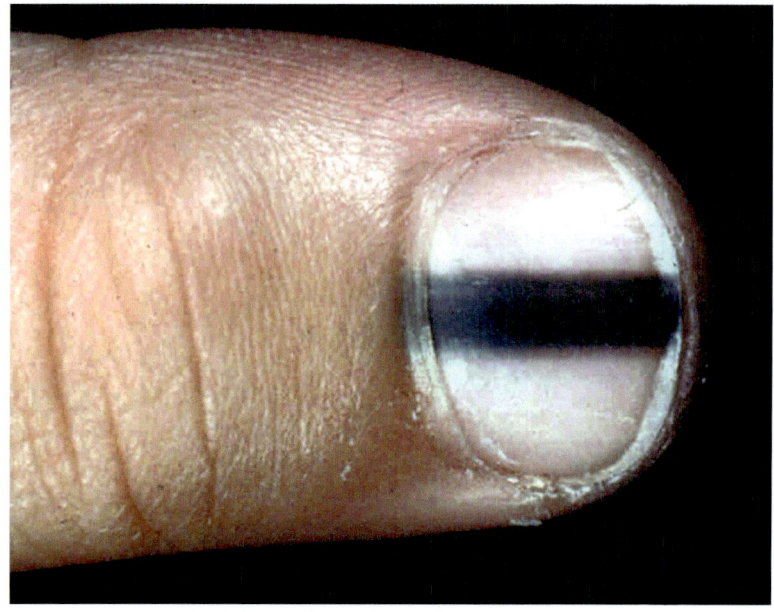

Figure 1.37 Pseudo-Hutchinson sign.

Benign lesions. Melanocytic nevus, nevoid melanosis.
Genetic. Peutz–Jeghers syndrome, congenital nevus.
Drug-related. Zidovudine, antimalarials, amlodipine, minocycline.
Other. Laugier–Hunziker disease, ethnic pigmentation, post-radiation, malnutrition, hematoma/trauma.

1.38 Koilonychia (Figure 1.38) is a thin, spoon-shaped (concave) nail deformity.[52]

Inflammatory. Alopecia areata, lichen planus, scleroderma, systemic lupus erythematosus, Raynaud's syndrome, psoriasis.
Infections. Syphilis, onychomycosis, scabies.
Systemic. Acanthosis nigricans, Plummer–Vinson syndrome, polycythemia vera, iron deficiency anemia, porphyria cutanea tarda, inflammatory bowel disease (IBD), celiac disease.

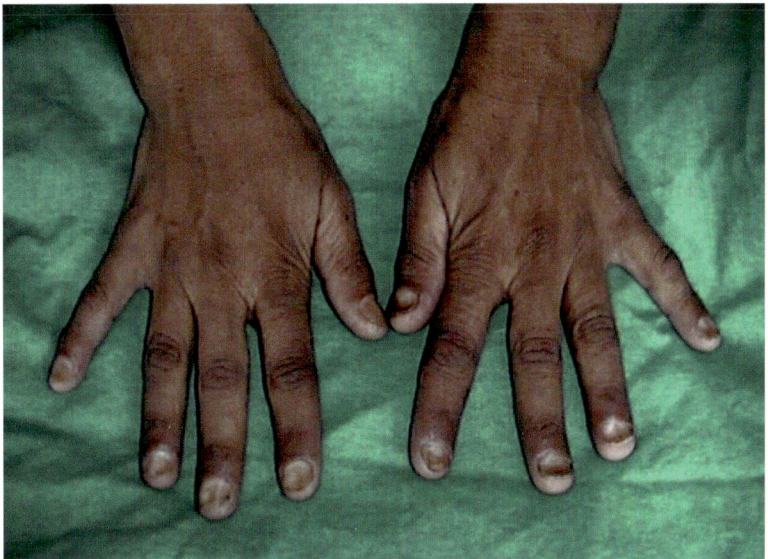

Figure 1.38 Koilonychia.

Genetic. Benign childhood koilonychia, familial koilonychia, mal de Meleda, Darier's disease, LEOPARD syndrome, incontinentia pigmenti, Goltz syndrome, nail-patella syndrome, ectodermal dysplasia, trichothiodystrophy, monilethrix, pachyonychia congenita, Cronkhite–Canada syndrome.
Trauma. Acrylic nail polishes, occupational causes.
Other. Coronary artery disease, high altitude, steatocystoma multiplex, idiopathic.

1.39 Nail pitting is characterized by small depressions or pits on the surface of the fingernails or toenails (Figure 1.39).[53]
Inflammatory. Pityriasis rosea, alopecia areata, eczema, psoriasis, lichen planus, sarcoidosis, perforating granuloma annulare, dermatitis of proximal nail fold, lichen nitidus, rheumatoid arthritis, dermatomyositis, reactive arthritis, contact eczema, pemphigus vulgaris, chronic kidney disease on dialysis, vitiligo, discoid lupus

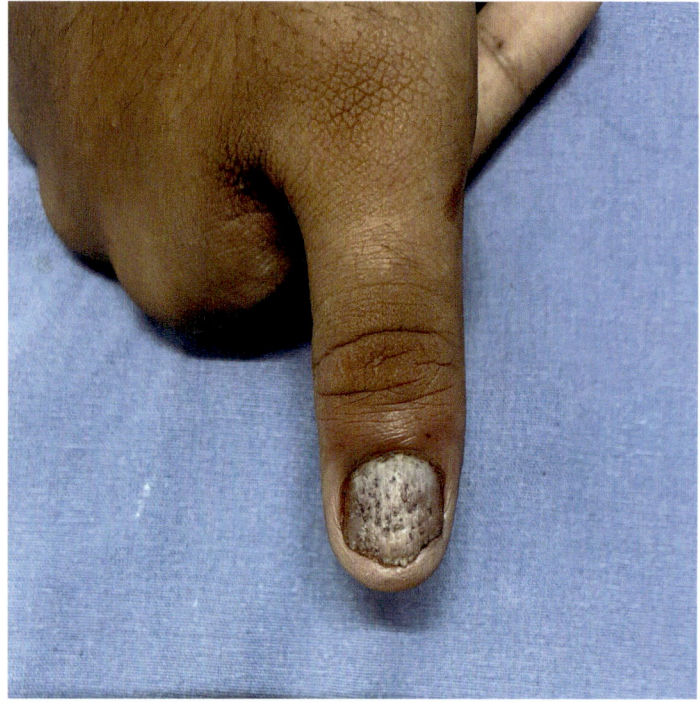

Figure 1.39 Nail pitting in psoriasis.

erythematosus, twenty-nail dystrophy (trachyonychia), parakeratosis pustulosa, osteoarthritis.
 Neoplasms. Histiocytosis.
 Infections. Onychomycosis, syphilis.
 Genetic. Myotonic dystrophy, incontinentia pigmenti, nail-patella syndrome, ectodermal dysplasia, Darier's disease.
 Other. Isotretinoin-induced, normal variant, trauma.

1.40 Palmar pits are punctiform depressions in the palms. They may be limited to the fingertips or involve both the palms and the palmar aspects of the fingers.[54]

Differential diagnoses by history and clinical features

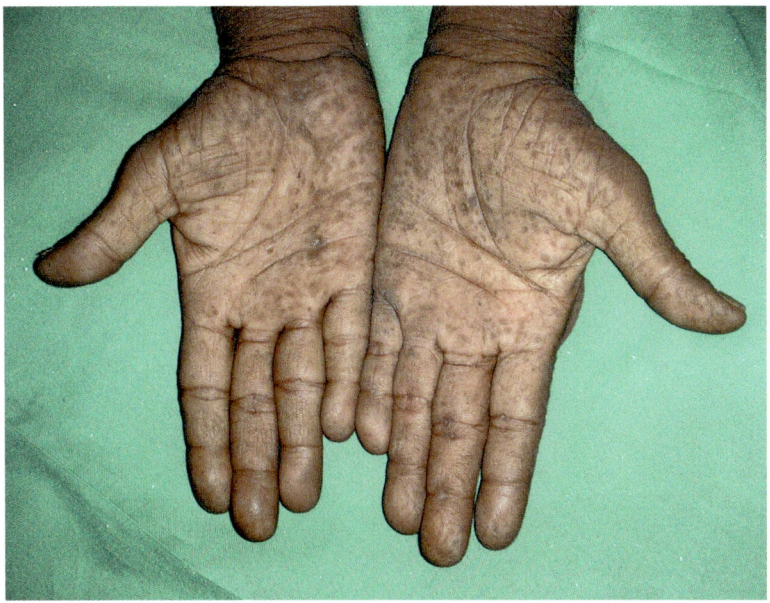

Figure 1.40 Palmar pits in Darier's disease.

Inflammatory. Lichen planus, lichen nitidus, systemic sclerosis, sarcoidosis, atopic eczema.

Infections. Viral warts, post-molluscum, pitted keratolysis.

Genetic. Gorlin syndrome, Darier's disease (Figure 1.40), Cowden syndrome, reticulate acropigmentation of Kitamura, punctate porokeratotic keratoderma, keratosis punctata palmoplantaris (Busche–Fisher–Bauer syndrome), Dowling–Degos syndrome.

Other. Arsenical keratosis, epidermodysplasia verruciformis, nevus comedonicus, chronic kidney failure, trichoepitheliomas, Dupuytren's contracture, paraneoplastic filiform hyperkeratosis.

Key points – differential diagnoses by history and clinical features

- Hypopigmentation tends to be more noticeable in people with darker skin, which in some instances can cause stigma and have serious psychological effects.
- Some dermatoses are readily identifiable from the shape, pattern, or distribution of the lesions.
- There are many skin conditions that mimic common dermatoses, such as acne and psoriasis.
- Examination of the palms and nails may provide useful clues to the diagnosis.

References

1. Basra MK, Shahrukh M. Burden of skin diseases. *Expert Rev Pharmacoecon Outcomes Res.* 2009;9(3):271-283.
2. Liu Y, Jain A, Eng C, et al. A deep learning system for differential diagnosis of skin diseases. *Nat Med.* 2020;26(6):900-908.
3. Krajnik M, Zylicz Z. Understanding pruritus in systemic disease. *J Pain Symptom Manage.* 2001;21(2):151-168.
4. Nawrocki S, Cha J. The etiology, diagnosis, and management of hyperhidrosis: a comprehensive review. *J Am Acad Dermatol.* 2019;81(3):657-666.
5. Schlossberg D. Fever and rash. *Infect Dis Clin North Am.* 1996;10(1):101-110.
6. Ghosh A, Das A, Sarkar R. Diffuse hyperpigmentation: a comprehensive approach. *Pigment Int.* 2018;5(1):4.
7. Speeckaert R, Van Gele M, Speeckaert MM, Lambert J, van Geel N. The biology of hyperpigmentation syndromes. *Pigment Cell Melanoma Res.* 2014;27(4):512-524.
8. Madireddy S, Crane JS. Hypopigmented macules. In: *StatPearls*. StatPearls Publishing, 2022. Last accessed 29 January 2023. ncbi.nlm.nih.gov/books/NBK563245
9. Saleem MD, Oussedik E, Picardo M, Schoch JJ. Acquired disorders with hypopigmentation: a clinical approach to diagnosis and treatment. *J Am Acad Dermatol.* 2019;80(5):1233-1250.e10.
10. Loomis CA. Linear hypopigmentation and hyperpigmentation, including mosaicism. *Semin Cutan Med Surg.* 1997;16(1):44-53.

11. van Geel N, Speeckaert M, Chevolet I, et al. Hypomelanoses in children. *J Cutan Aesthet Surg*. 2013;6(2):65-72.
12. Bhalla M, Garg S. Acral melanosis. *Pigment Int*. 2018;5:14-27.
13. Zhang J, Li M, Yao Z. Updated review of genetic reticulate pigmentary disorders. *Br J Dermatol*. 2017;177(4):945-959.
14. Sreeja C, Ramakrishnan K, Vijayalakshmi D, Devi M, Aesha I, Vijayabanu B. Oral pigmentation: a review. *J Pharm Bioallied Sci*. 2015;7(Suppl 2):S403-S408.
15. Kumarasinghe P, Hewitt D. Neoplasms with pigmentary changes or discoloration. In: Lahiri K, Chatterjee M, Sarkar R, eds. *Pigmentary Disorders. A Comprehensive Compendium*. Jaypee Brothers Medical Publishers Ltd; 2014:95-96.
16. Cunliffe WJ, Holland DB, Jeremy A. Comedone formation: etiology, clinical presentation, and treatment. *Clin Dermatol*. 2004;22(5):367-374.
17. Fernandes-Flores A. Lesions with an epidermal hyperplastic pattern: morphologic clues in the differential diagnosis. *Am J Dermatopathol*. 2016;38(1):1-16.
18. Zhao CY, Murrell DF. Blistering diseases in neonates. *Curr Opin Pediatr*. 2016;28(4):500-506.
19. Mengesha YM, Bennett ML. Pustular skin disorders: diagnosis and treatment. *Am J Clin Dermatol*. 2002;3(6):389-400.
20. Freitas E, Rodrigues MA, Torres T. Diagnosis, screening and treatment of patients with palmoplantar pustulosis (PPP): a review of current practices and recommendations. *Clin Cosmet Investig Dermatol*. 2020;13:561-578.
21. Obeid G, Do G, Kirby L, Hughes C, Sbidian E, Le Cleach L. Interventions for chronic palmoplantar pustulosis. *Cochrane Database Syst Rev*. 2020;1(1):CD011628.
22. Bubna AK. Umbilicated lesions in dermatology. *Clin Dermatol Rev*. 2019;3(1):99.
23. Diociaiuti A, Cutrone M, Rotunno R, et al. Angioma serpiginosum: a case report and review of the literature. *Ital J Pediatr*. 2019;45(1):1-5.
24. Narayanasetty NK, Pai VV, Athanikar SB. Annular lesions in dermatology. *Indian J Dermatol*. 2013;58(2):157.
25. Tierney EP, Badger J. Etiology and pathogenesis of necrolytic migratory erythema: review of the literature. *MedGenMed*. 2004;6(3):4.
26. Malvankar DD, Sacchidanand S, Mallikarjun M, Nataraj HV. Linear lesions in dermatology. *Indian J Dermatol Venereol Leprol*. 2011;77(6):722-726.
27. Senner S, Eicher L, Nasifoglu S, Wollenberg A. Linear patterns of the skin and their dermatoses. *J Dtsch Dermatol Ges*. 2020;18(4):341-364.

28. Chairatchaneeboon M, Thanomkitti K, Kim EJ. Parapsoriasis – a diagnosis with an identity crisis: a narrative review. *Dermatol Ther (Heidelb)*. 2022;12(5):1091-1102.
29. Hu CH, Winkelmann RK. Digitate dermatosis: a new look at symmetrical, small plaque parapsoriasis. *Archiv Dermatol*. 1973;107(1):65-69.
30. Drago F, Ciccarese G, Parodi A. Pityriasis rosea and pityriasis rosea-like eruptions: how to distinguish them? *JAAD Case Rep*. 2018;4(8):800-801.
31. Urbina F, Das A, Sudy E. Clinical variants of pityriasis rosea. *World J Clin Cases*. 2017;5(6):203-211.
32. Tirado-Sánchez A, Bonifaz A. Nodular lymphangitis (sporotrichoid lymphocutaneous infections). Clues to differential diagnosis. *J Fungi (Basel)*. 2018;4(2):56.
33. el Hayderi L, Libon F, Tassoudji NN, Rübben A, Dezfoulian B, Nikkels AF. Zosteriform dermatoses – a review. *Glob Dermatol*. 2015;2(4):163-173.
34. Ergun T. Pathergy phenomenon. *Front Med (Lausanne)*. 2021;8:639404.
35. Sequeira FF, Daryani D. The oral and skin pathergy test. *Indian J Dermatol Venereol Leprol*. 2011;77:526.
36. Patterson JW. The perforating disorders. *J Am Acad Dermatol*. 1984;10(4):561-581.
37. Harbaoui S, Litaiem N. Acquired perforating dermatosis. In: *StatPearls*. StatPearls Publishing; 2023. Last accessed 19 April 2023. ncbi.nlm.nih.gov/books/NBK539715
38. Tziotzios C, Lee JYW, Brier T, et al. Lichen planus and lichenoid dermatoses. *J Am Acad Dermatol*. 2018;79(5):789-804.
39. Wick MR. Psoriasiform dermatitides: a brief review. *Semin Diagn Pathol*. 2017;34(3):220-225.
40. Davis EC, Callender VD. A review of acne in ethnic skin. *J Clin Aesthet Dermatol*. 2010;3(4):24-38.
41. Nair PA, Salazar FJ. Acneiform eruptions. In: *StatPearls*. StatPearls Publishing; 2023. Last accessed 24 April 2023. ncbi.nlm.nih.gov/books/NBK459207
42. Plewig G, Jansen T. Acneiform dermatoses. *Dermatology* 1998;196(1):102-107.
43. Ashourian N, Mousdicas N. Pellagra-like dermatitis. *N Engl J Med*. 2006;354(15):1614.
44. Hendricks WM. Pellagra and pellagra like dermatoses: etiology, differential diagnosis, dermatopathology, and treatment. *Semin Dermatol*. 1991;10(4):282-292.
45. Regan TD, Norton SA. The scarring mechanism of smallpox. *J Am Acad Dermatol*. 2004;50(4):591-594.
46. Chantorn R, Lim HW, Shwayder TA. Photosensitivity disorders in children: Part I. *J Am Acad Dermatol*. 2012;67(6):1093.e1-1093.e18.

47. Chantorn R, Lim HW, Shwayder TA. Photosensitivity disorders in children: Part II. *J Am Acad Dermatol.* 2012;67(6):1113.e1-1113.e15.
48. Brown DN, Wieser I, Wang C, Dabaja BS, Duvic M. Leonine facies (LF) and mycosis fungoides (MF): a single-center study and systematic review of the literature. *J Am Acad Dermatol.* 2015;73(6):976-986.
49. Kumar A, Karthikeyan K. Madarosis: a marker of many maladies. *Int J Trichology.* 2012;4(1):3-18.
50. Sand M, Sand D, Brors D, Altmeyer P, Mann B, Bechara FG. Cutaneous lesions of the external ear. *Head Face Med.* 2008;4(1):1-13.
51. Baran R, Kechijian P. Hutchinson's sign: a reappraisal. *J Am Acad Dermatol.* 1996;34(1):87-90.
52. Walker J, Baran R, Vélez N, Jellinek N. Koilonychia: an update on pathophysiology, differential diagnosis and clinical relevance. *J Eur Acad Dermatol Venereol.* 2016;30(11):1985-1991.
53. Jadhav VM, Mahajan PM, Mhaske CB. Nail pitting and onycholysis. *Indian J Dermatol Venereol Leprol.* 2009;75:631.
54. Adya KA, Inamadar AC, Palit A. "Pitted" lesions in dermatology. *Int J Dermatol.* 2017;56(1):3-17.

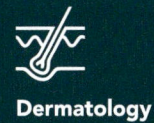

Dermatology

2 Refining the differential diagnosis with investigations and tests

- 2.1 Syphilis (VDRL blood test) *60*
- 2.2 Vitamin D deficiency (blood test) *61*
- 2.3 Eosinophilia (blood test) *61*
- 2.4 Eosinophilic spongiosis (histology) *63*
- 2.5 Infectious granulomas (histology) *63*
- 2.6 Splendore-Hoeppli phenomenon (histology) *65*
- 2.7 Pseudoepitheliomatous hyperplasia (histology) *66*
- 2.8 Allergic contact dermatitis (patch testing) *67*

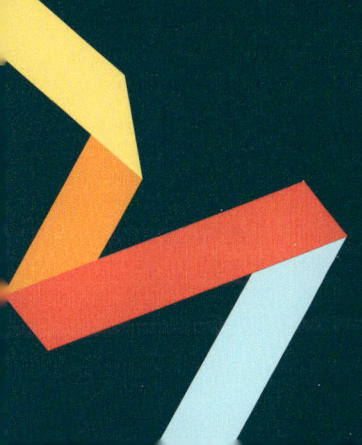

HEALTHCARE

The lists of potential diagnoses based on clinical signs and symptoms in Chapter 1 provide the non-specialist with a differential diagnosis for a wide range of dermatoses in people with skin of color (SOC), some of which may not have been previously considered. As the diagnostic work-up continues with various tests, the list may be refined to a narrower set of differential diagnoses or even a single diagnosis.

While diagnostic certainty is not always needed to start treatment, further investigations may be required to rule out conflicting or potentially dangerous conditions. For example, if the list of differential diagnoses includes eczema and tinea infection, a topical corticosteroid may be considered for the eczema; however, this could worsen a tinea infection. It may, therefore, be prudent to test for fungal infection before starting treatment. If there was suspicion of malignancy, a biopsy would be essential.

Investigations and tests

Skin swabs can be taken when bacterial or viral infections are suspected. It is important to use the correct swab as different transport mediums are used for bacterial and viral cultures. To collect the specimen, the tip of the swab is rubbed over the suspect area.

Skin scrapings are taken to confirm fungal infection. Loose skin scales are collected with the blunt edge of a scalpel, ideally from the scaly edge of the lesion where a higher yield of active microorganisms can be retrieved.

Nail clippings and extracted hair can be examined by direct microscopy before being plated for fungal culture.

Slit skin smears are performed to detect infections such as leprosy and leishmaniasis. A slit skin smear involves making a small superficial incision in the skin (usually from the infiltrated plaque), ensuring no blood is drawn. The tissue fluid from the cut is smeared on a glass slide, stained, and examined for microorganisms.

Blood tests help to identify inflammation, systemic disease, infection, and nutritional deficiencies. For example, raised eosinophil levels may indicate an allergic skin disease, while elevated neutrophil levels may indicate infection or inflammation. Specific serology should be requested when there is suspicion of infection.

Biopsy enables histological evaluation, which is particularly important when there is suspicion of malignancy or when an inflammatory dermatosis needs to be confirmed. Procedures include shave biopsy in which the portion of the lesion above the surface of the skin is scraped to gather a cell sample, punch biopsy in which a small core of skin (including deeper levels) is sampled, and excisional biopsy in which the entire lesion along with a margin of healthy skin is removed.

Patch testing is used to evaluate allergic contact dermatitis. Suspect chemicals are applied on small discs that are secured to the patient's back by strips of tape. These are left in place on unaffected clear skin for 48 hours to provoke a reaction, which reveals culprit allergens.

Wood's light examination. The handheld Wood's lamp emits ultraviolet (UV) A light, under which healthy skin appears slightly blue; white spots indicate thicker skin, yellow spots indicate oily patches, and purple spots indicate dryness. It can detect areas of hyper- or hypopigmented skin and fluorescence that indicates a fungal, bacterial, or parasitic infection. The lamp must be used in a completely dark room on clean skin, and both patient and clinician need to protect their eyes.

Dermatoscopy. A handheld dermatoscope has a high-magnification lens and inbuilt illuminating system that enables examination of subsurface skin structures in the epidermis, dermo-epidermal junction, and upper dermis that are not visible to the naked eye. It may be useful to help diagnose inflammatory and pigmentary dermatoses, infections, and disorders of the hair, nails, and scalp.

Radiological imaging by CT, MRI, ultrasonography, or radiography is not routinely used in dermatology, but may be required to investigate systemic symptoms, and is essential for staging advanced melanoma.

Interpreting diagnostic tests

When interpreting test results, clinicians must consider the specificity of the test, that is, its ability to identify a specific disease. Many dermatological tests can help to refine the differential diagnosis, but not all provide a definitive diagnosis. Examples are given below.

Blood tests can help identify underlying conditions that cause a skin problem: for example, an inflammatory condition or infection.

2.1 Syphilis. The Venereal Disease Research Laboratory (VDRL) test is one of several non-treponemal tests used to screen for syphilis. Although it detects antibodies to syphilis (syphilis reagin), it is not specific for the disease, and other conditions that may render a positive VDRL test should be considered.[1]

Infections. Syphilis (Figure 2.1), lepromatous leprosy, infectious mononucleosis, malaria, leptospirosis, borreliosis, endemic treponematoses.

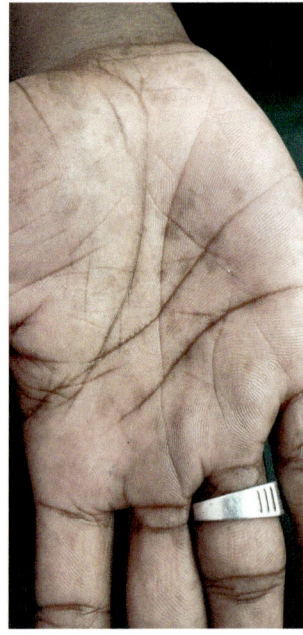

Figure 2.1 A maculopapular rash on the palms and soles is a hallmark feature of secondary syphilis.

Physiological. Pregnancy, idiopathic.

Inflammatory. Antiphospholipid syndrome, systemic lupus erythematosus.

Other causes. Drug abuse, lymphoma, cirrhosis.

2.2 Vitamin D deficiency. Vitamin D levels are best determined by measuring the concentration of 25-hydroxyvitamin D in blood. While the association between vitamin D deficiency and psoriasis has been well established,[2] studies have also shown that decreased levels of 25-hydroxyvitamin D are likely to be a contributing factor in the development of other skin diseases.[3,4] Conditions associated with low vitamin D levels are listed below.

Inflammatory. Psoriasis (Figure 2.2), atopic eczema, pemphigoid, pemphigus, vitiligo, acne.

Congenital. Ichthyosis.

Neoplasms. Malignant melanoma, non-melanoma skin cancer.

Other. Female pattern hair thinning, telogen effluvium.

2.3 Eosinophilia is a common finding in a wide range of skin diseases, including allergic reactions and neoplastic processes, but it is not pathognomonic for any specific dermatosis.[5]

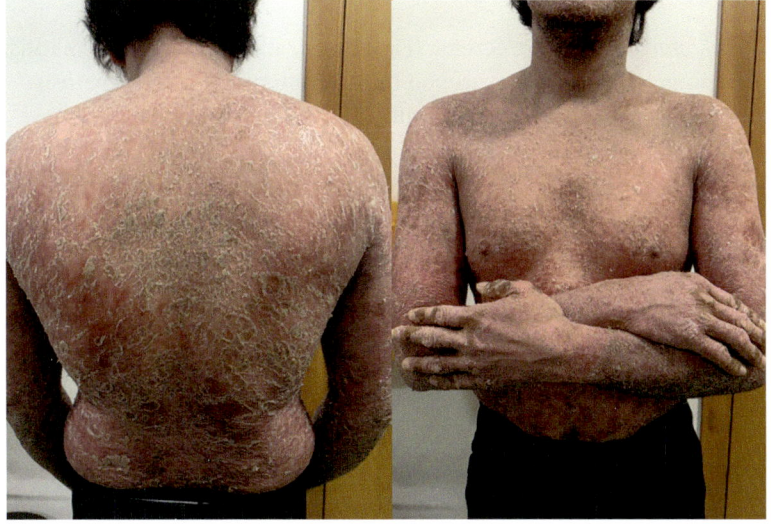

Figure 2.2 Erythrodermic psoriasis in a patient with vitamin D deficiency.

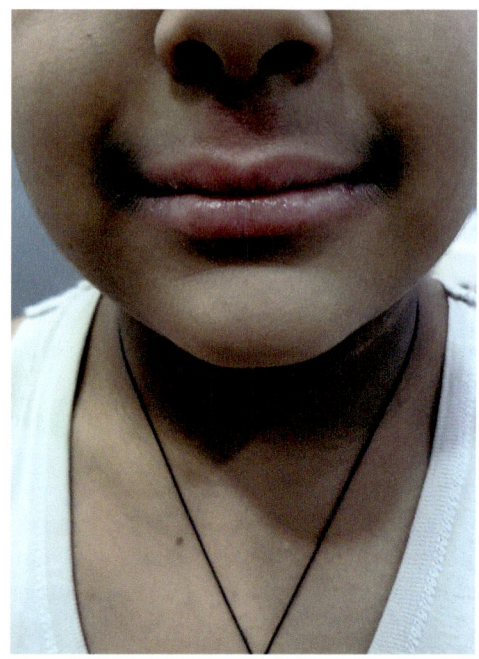

Figure 2.3 Atopic eczema.

Inflammatory. Atopic eczema (Figure 2.3), allergic contact dermatitis, pemphigoid, urticaria, arthropod bites, eosinophilic granulomatosis with polyangiitis, eosinophilic cellulitis (Wells' syndrome), eosinophilic fasciitis, eosinophilic pustular folliculitis, infantile hypereosinophilic syndrome, angiolymphoid hyperplasia with eosinophilia, systemic lupus erythematosus, dermatitis herpetiformis, DRESS syndrome and other drug-related reactions, eosinophilic annular erythema.

Infections. Parasitic diseases (including scabies, loiasis, and schistosomiasis), HIV infection, coccidioidomycosis.

Neoplasms. Lymphomas, leukemias, mastocytosis.

Other. Hyper-immunoglobulin (Ig) E syndrome, Omenn syndrome, eosinophilia-myalgia syndrome, idiopathic hypereosinophilic syndrome.

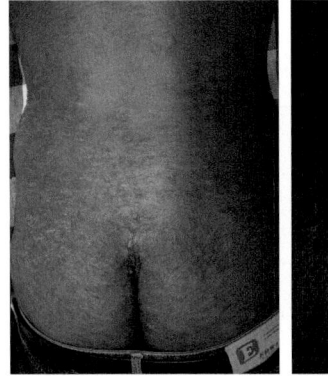 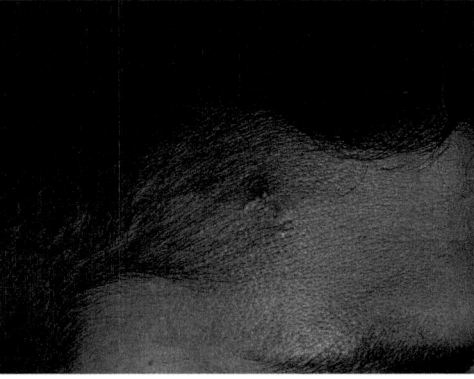

Figure 2.4 Extensive larva migrans infection, with cutaneous presentation at different locations in the same patient.

Histopathology. While histological analysis can help to refine the list of differential diagnoses by providing information about the disease process (for example, inflammatory versus neoplastic), the information can be non-specific. However, in some instances, the use of specific stains helps to identify the causative agent or organism.

2.4 Eosinophilic spongiosis is a histological feature shared by many different disorders characterized by intraepidermal eosinophils associated with spongiosis.[6]

Inflammatory. Bullous pemphigoid, pemphigus and its variants, subcorneal pustular dermatosis, dermatitis herpetiformis, eosinophilic cellulitis, photoallergic reaction, allergic contact dermatitis, eosinophilic folliculitis, herpes gestationis.

Infections. Scabies, milker's nodules, parasitic infection (larva migrans) (Figure 2.4).

Genetic. Incontinentia pigmenti, Job's syndrome (hypereosinophilic syndrome).

Other. Arthropod reactions, drug reactions, erythema toxicum neonatorum.

2.5 Infectious granulomas. Granulomatous inflammation is caused by a variety of bacterial, fungal, and parasitic infections. Histologically, 50% of the infiltrate of granulomas is made up of histiocytes (macrophages) (Figure 2.5).

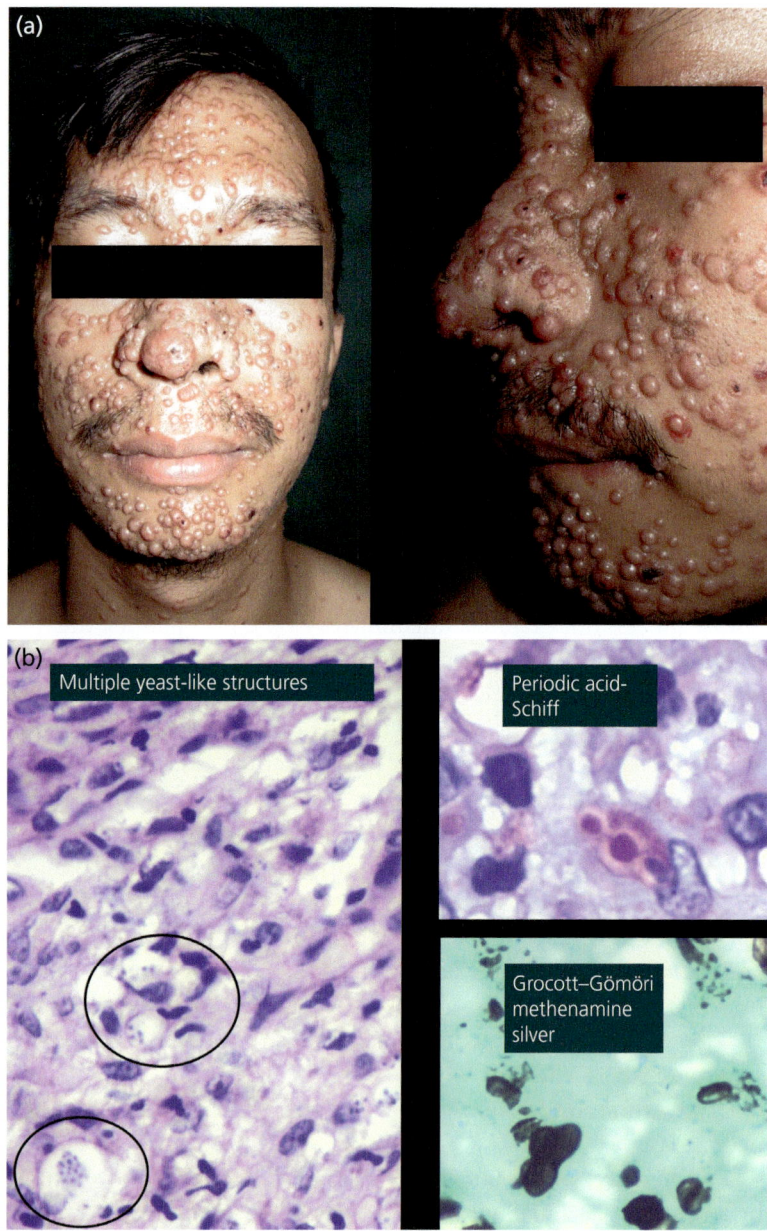

Figure 2.5 (a) Clinical and (b) histological presentation of histoplasmosis.

Careful examination of initial histology can reveal organisms within the histiocytes, but special tissue stains are required to further identify the causative organism. For example, *Leishmania* parasites can be identified by Giemsa staining, *Mycobacterium leprae* (causing leprosy) require Fite-Faraco stain, and fungal infections stain with Grocott–Gömöri methenamine silver (GMS), Ziehl-Neelsen (acid-fast stain), or periodic acid-Schiff stains (see Figure 2.5).[7]

Bacterial. Lepromatous leprosy, granuloma inguinale, lymphogranuloma venereum, rhinoscleroma.

Fungal. Cryptococcosis, histoplasmosis (see Figure 2.5), talaromycosis.

Parasitic. Leishmaniasis, Chagas disease (*Trypanosoma cruzi*), schistosomiasis.

2.6 Splendore-Hoeppli phenomenon is a morphologically unique inflammatory process characterized by bright eosinophilic material radiating out around infectious microorganisms or necrotic material (Figure 2.6a).[8] It comprises an antigen–antibody complex, tissue debris, and fibrosis. However, it is not specific, as it has been observed in several fungal, bacterial, and parasitic infections.

Fungal. Sporotrichosis, zygomycosis, candidiasis, aspergillosis, blastomycosis, eumycetoma (Figure 2.6b), Majocchi's granuloma, *Pityrosporum* folliculitis.

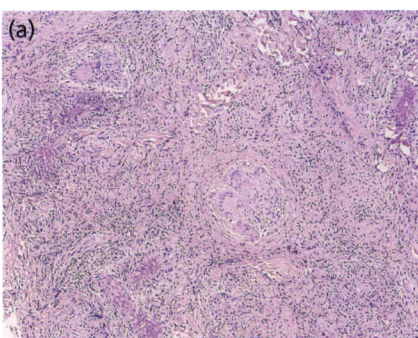
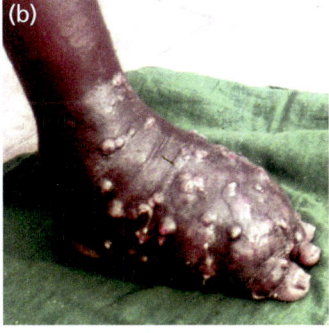

Figure 2.6 Splendore-Hoeppli phenomenon. (a) Histology showing eosinophilic material consisting of immunoglobulin and cell debris radiating out from entomophthoromycosis. Image reproduced courtesy of Dr Meenakshi Batrani, Consultant Dermatopathologist, Delhi Dermpath Laboratory, New Delhi, India. (b) Eumycetoma is a chronic deep fungal infection of the skin and subcutaneous tissue that most commonly affects the feet.

Bacterial. Botryomycosis, nocardiosis, actinomycosis.

Parasitic. Strongyloides, schistosomiasis, cutaneous larva migrans, orbital pythiosis.

Non-infective. Hypereosinophilic syndrome, allergic conjunctival granuloma, squamous cell carcinoma, silk suture reaction.

2.7 Pseudoepitheliomatous hyperplasia is a reactive change to the epidermis characterized by hyperplasia and an increase in adnexal structures. It is prominent in several inflammatory, infectious, and neoplastic skin conditions.[9]

Inflammatory. Hypertrophic lichen planus, pemphigus vegetans, pyoderma gangrenosum, prurigo nodularis (Figure 2.7), lichen sclerosus, verrucous lupus erythematosus, chondrodermatis nodularis helicis, lichen simplex chronicus.

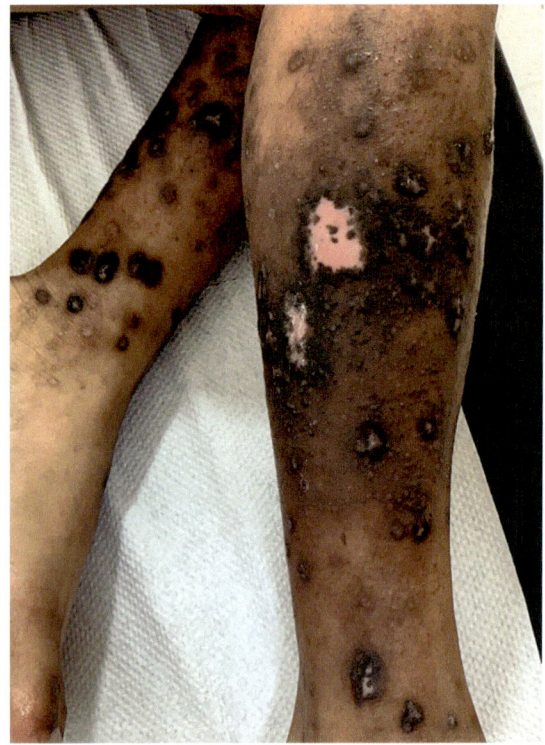

Figure 2.7 Prurigo nodularis on the extensor surfaces of the lower legs.

Infections. Mycobacteria, syphilis, viral warts, blastomycosis, chromoblastomycosis, sporotrichosis, orf.
Vascular. Venous stasis ulcer, chronic ulcer, severe lymphedema.
Neoplasms. Keratoacanthoma, squamous cell carcinoma, basal cell carcinoma, granular cell tumor, melanoma, cutaneous T-cell lymphoma.
Trauma. Borders of healing wounds, previous biopsy site, tattoo, arthropod bite, urostomy and colostomy sites.
Other. Halogenoderma.

Patch testing. Interpretation of patch testing in patients with SOC can be difficult, as positive tests present with lichenification and hyperpigmentation, rather than erythema and vesicles. The usual bright red or pink hues for positive results may appear violaceous, black, or faint pink. In patients with very heavily pigmented skin, erythema may be too subtle to appreciate. As a result, there may be more false negatives when patch testing on SOC compared with white skin. Using light with a 45–90° angle to identify features like papules and vesicles is advisable. A geometric raised plaque could also be considered a positive reaction.[10,11]

2.8 Allergic contact dermatitis can occur in up to 20% of the population. However, information regarding the common allergens that cause contact dermatitis in SOC is limited. A recent review suggests that the most common positive reactions in African American people are to paraphenylenediamine (PPD) (Figure 2.8), balsam of Peru, bacitracin, fragrance mix, and nickel. In Hispanic people, the most common positives are carba mix, nickel, and thiuram mix. In Asian people, nickel, fragrance mix, and potassium dichromate give the most common positive reactions.[10]

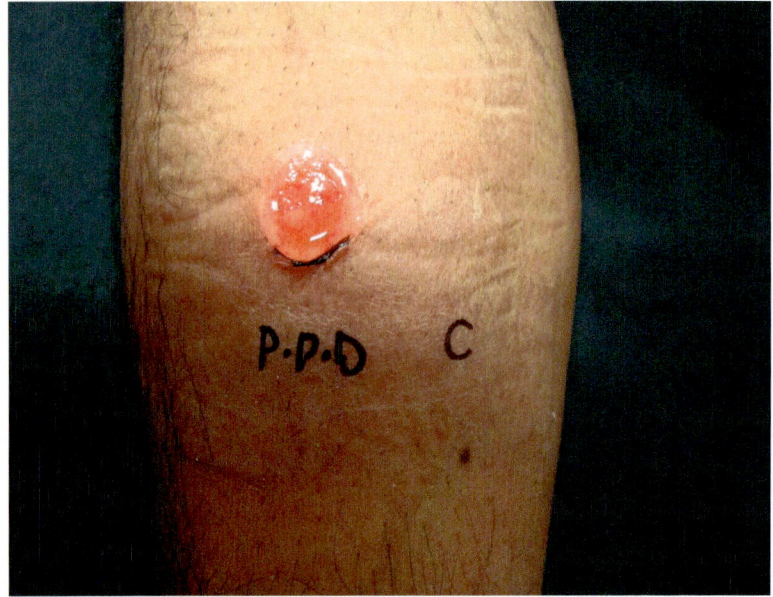

Figure 2.8 Violent reaction to paraphenylenediamine (PPD), a chemical that is widely used as a permanent hair dye, on patch testing.

Key points – refining the differential diagnosis with investigations and tests

- An initial differential diagnosis based on clinical features can be further refined with dermatological tests, including microbiological evaluation from skin swabs and scrapings, blood tests, histological analysis of biopsies, and patch testing.
- Blood tests may not be diagnostic but can provide clues toward the final diagnosis.
- While histological analysis is often non-specific, special stains can help to identify bacterial, fungal, and parasitic organisms that cause granulomatous inflammation.
- Slit skin smears are useful to diagnose chronic infections such as leprosy or leishmaniasis.
- It can be difficult to interpret patch testing in patients with SOC as positive tests often present with hyperpigmentation rather than erythema and vesicles, and any erythema may be too subtle to appreciate.
- There are likely to be more false negatives when patch testing patients with SOC than those with fair skin.

References

1. Nayak S, Acharjya B. VDRL test and its interpretation. *Indian J Dermatol.* 2012;57(1):3-8.
2. Barrea L, Savanelli MC, Di Somma C, et al. Vitamin D and its role in psoriasis: an overview of the dermatologist and nutritionist. *Rev Endocr Metab Disord.* 2017;18(2):195-205.
3. Umar M, Sastry KS, Al Ali F, Al-Khulaifi M, Wang E, Chouchane AI. Vitamin D and the pathophysiology of inflammatory skin diseases. *Skin Pharmacol Physiol.* 2018;31(2):74-86.
4. Wadhwa B, Relhan V, Goel K, Kochhar AM, Garg VK. Vitamin D and skin diseases: a review. *Indian J Dermatol Venereol Leprol.* 2015;81(4):344.
5. Radonjic-Hoesli S, Brüggen MC, Feldmeyer L, Simon HU, Simon D. Eosinophils in skin diseases. *Semin Immunopathol.* 2021;43(3):393-409.
6. Morais KL, Miyamoto D, Maruta CW, Aoki V. Diagnostic approach of eosinophilic spongiosis. *An Bras Dermatol.* 2019;94(6):724-728.

7. Shah KK, Pritt BS, Alexander MP. Histopathologic review of granulomatous inflammation. *J Clin Tuberc Other Mycobact Dis*. 2017;7:1-12.
8. Hussein MR. Mucocutaneous Splendore-Hoeppli phenomenon. *J Cutan Pathol*. 2008;35(11):979-988.
9. Zayour M, Lazova R. Pseudoepitheliomatous hyperplasia: a review. *Am J Dermatopathol*. 2011;33(2):112-122; quiz 123-126.
10. Burli A, Vashi NA, Li BS, Maibach HI. Allergic contact dermatitis and patch testing in skin of color patients. *Dermatitis*. 2023;34(2):85-89.
11. Tamazian S, Oboite M, Treat JR. Patch testing in skin of color: a brief report. *Pediatr Dermatol*. 2021;38(4):952-953.

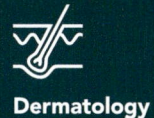

3 Presentation and management of common dermatoses in skin of color

3.1 Acne *72*
3.2 Eczema *74*
3.3 Psoriasis *77*
3.4 Hidradenitis suppurativa *78*
3.5 Post-inflammatory hyperpigmentation *80*
3.6 Skin cancer *81*
3.7 Psychological factors *87*

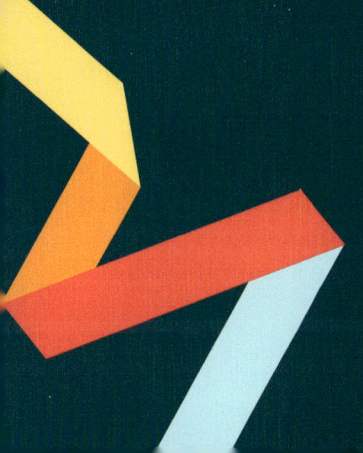

HEALTHCARE

The skin manifestations of common dermatoses, such as acne, eczema, and psoriasis, are different in skin of color (SOC) than in lighter skin tones. Clinicians need to be familiar with these differences to make a timely and accurate diagnosis, which in many instances is important for reducing morbidity and mortality.

3.1 Acne

Acne is one of the most common inflammatory conditions in people with SOC. In one study of female patients only, acne vulgaris was found to be most prevalent in African American or Hispanic people (37% and 32%, respectively), followed by Asian (30%), White (24%), and Continental Indian (23%) people. Individuals of Asian descent were found to have a higher number of inflammatory lesions than comedonal lesions (20% vs 10%).[1]

Clinical presentation is variable. Comedones evolve into papules, then pustules and cysts. Seborrhea is also common. There may be specific triggers. For example, the use of hair oils can cause pomade acne in which comedones develop along the hairline, and skin-lightening products may contain potent topical steroids that increase comedogenesis. The imbalance of hormones associated with polycystic ovary syndrome (PCOS), which presents at a younger age and with normal body mass index in women of South East Asian background,[2] can also cause acne.

Post-inflammatory hyperpigmentation (PIH) and keloids are long-term complications that are more likely to occur in SOC. The psychological effects of PIH can be more detrimental than the acne itself.

Management. Early and effective treatment is the most important management principle, as it prevents PIH and keloidal scarring.[3] Daily sunscreen use also reduces the intensity of PIH (see pages 85–86).

Topical treatment. Adapalene, a second-generation topical retinoid, reduces potential irritation and may help address PIH as well. Tazarotene is another retinoid that could be considered. It is available as a cream, which is better tolerated than gel. Combining a retinoid at night with topical azelaic acid in the morning is also very helpful as azelaic acid has a beneficial effect on PIH.[4]

Systemic treatment should also be started early if there is no response to topical medications.[4] Oral antibiotics that have antibacterial and anti-inflammatory actions should be used, including tetracyclines, erythromycin, and trimethoprim. Early low-dose isotretinoin can be effective in bringing about complete early remission. Isotretinoin is useful for treating nodulocystic acne (Figure 3.1) and acne that is resistant to topical therapy or oral antibiotics, and it can improve PIH.

Another useful oral agent in post-teen acne in SOC is spironolactone, which can be considered in female patients who do not respond to isotretinoin.

Laser treatment of acne scarring. Scarring following acne can affect 95% of people with the condition.[5] The severity of scarring increases with prolonged inflammation. Prompt treatment of active acne is therefore essential. The goal of laser treatment is to improve the appearance of scarring with minimal side effects.

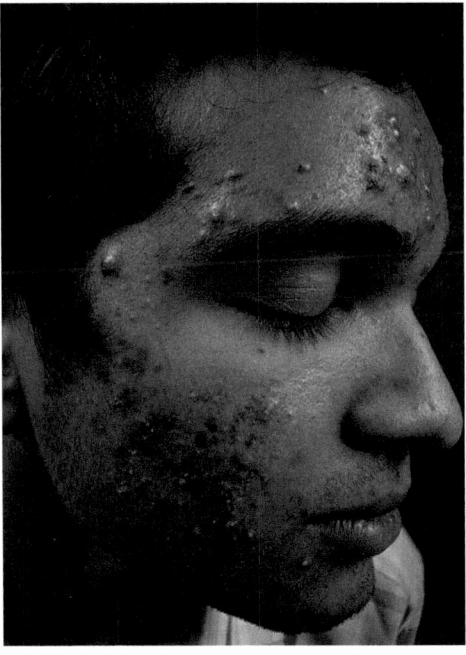

Figure 3.1 Nodulocystic acne.

Ablative lasers like carbon dioxide (CO_2) and erbium:yttrium-aluminum-garnett (YAG) are clinically effective and require only one treatment. CO_2 lasers produce more coagulation and thereby predispose to more hyperpigmentation, but this may stimulate collagen deposition and therefore improve outcomes. Risks include pain, infection, erythema, PIH/hypopigmentation, and scarring.

Pulsed dye laser therapy is effective for erythematous and hypertrophic scars. It targets blood vessels, causing local ischemia followed by new collagen formation. Laser settings with lower fluences are required for darker skin types. Purpura and PIH are potential side effects.

Test patches are recommended before full treatment in patients with SOC. This helps clinicians provide the most effective dosage while minimizing the risk of PIH. The typical site for patch testing is the pre-auricular area. Priming the skin with ultraviolet (UV) photoprotection, skin-lightening agents, and chemical peels before laser therapy reduces the risk of PIH.

Patients should be provided with realistic expectations as no treatment will eliminate scarring.

3.2 Eczema

The incidence of eczema (atopic dermatitis) is higher in people with SOC than those with fair skin, with Black children being twice as likely to develop atopic eczema as White children.[6]

Clinical presentation. Morphologically, eczema can appear with follicular, prurigo-like, or lichenified characteristics. Pityriasis alba is more prevalent in Indian children with eczema. Other manifestations like pigmentation in the neck (atopic neck) (Figure 3.2a) or infraorbital skin folds (Dennie–Morgan folds) and increased skin markings on the palms (hyperlinear palms) are more common in SOC.

In the subacute phase, eczema presents as areas of erythematous, itchy, dry skin, progressing to weeping papules and blisters in the acute phase. It should be noted that erythema in SOC may present as shades of violet or an increase in pigmentation leading to a darkening of the skin. In the chronic phase, the skin may appear psoriasiform, scaly, or lichenoid. Hyperpigmentation is common in both the acute and chronic phases in SOC, and PIH may persist for many months.

Presentation and management of common dermatoses in skin of color

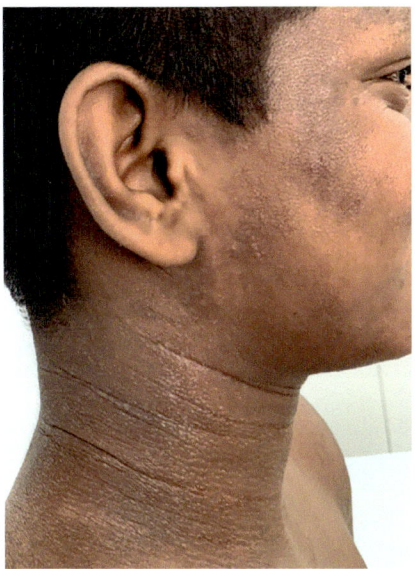

Figure 3.2a Atopic dermatitis on the face and neck.

Asian individuals tend to present with well-demarcated lesions with more scaling and lichenification than White individuals. Eczema typically has a flexural presentation, but in Black people it often presents as distinct papules on the extensors and trunk.[6,7]

Structurally, black skin is considered to have a lower ratio of ceramides to cholesterol in the stratum corneum and higher transepidermal water loss, causing dry skin and more severe eczema than in white skin.

Management. The severity of eczema is usually underestimated in SOC and therefore treatment is often suboptimal. Current treatment guidelines are similar across all skin types.

Topical treatment. Humectant moisturizers like urea, glycerin, and propylene glycol can cause irritation in patients with sensitive SOC. Bland emollients are therefore essential and need to be applied as often as possible.

Topical steroids are the mainstay of treatment. However, the high potency of topical steroids can cause hypopigmentation of darker skin.

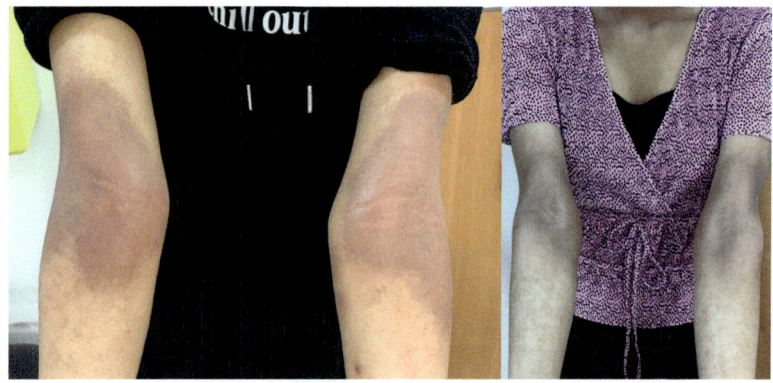

Figure 3.2b Before (left) and after (right) treatment of eczema with a Janus kinase inhibitor.

Topical calcineurin inhibitors (tacrolimus, pimecrolimus) have similar efficacy in SOC as in white skin.

Phototherapy should be considered for individuals with more widespread eczema. Narrowband UVB requires greater doses in more pigmented skin types. However, dyspigmentation may occur after this therapy.

Systemic treatment. Effective agents include methotrexate, ciclosporin, mycophenolate, and azathioprine. One study showed that the oral bioavailability of ciclosporin in Black patients may be 20–50% lower than in White people.[8] Higher doses of ciclosporin may therefore be needed. Dupilumab, an interleukin (IL)-4 and -13 inhibitor, has demonstrated efficacy in improving quality of life in people with SOC. IL-13 inhibitors (tralokinumab, lebrikizumab) and Janus kinase inhibitors (baricitinib, abrocitinib, upadacitinib), which target the JAK-STAT signaling cascade, have also shown efficacy in atopic dermatitis but ethnicity data are limited (Figure 3.2b).

3.3 Psoriasis

Psoriasis is reported more commonly in white skin, but the condition may be under-reported and underestimated in SOC.[9]

Clinical presentation. In white skin, erythema in psoriatic plaques is usually described as pink with an overlying silver scale. This manifests as less conspicuous violaceous or hyperpigmented skin in SOC, which can cause diagnostic challenges as active psoriasis can be mistaken for PIH. The plaques are usually well demarcated and often distributed over extensor surfaces, particularly the elbows and knees, and the scalp. Plaques have been found to be thicker and may be more extensive in people of African American descent due to delayed diagnosis.[9] Plaques have been reported to be smaller and less widespread in East Asian patients despite higher expression of the IL-17 and IL-17A proinflammatory cytokines.[10]

Management

Topical treatment. Topical steroids can induce hypopigmentation in SOC. For topical scalp treatment, therapy may need to be individualized according to hair texture, washing frequency, and styling practices.

Phototherapy is effective in those with darker skin color, but higher doses may be needed. The disadvantage is temporary darkening of skin, which is undesirable for some patients with SOC. It can temporarily aggravate psoriasis-induced pigmentation.

Systemic treatment. Current psoriasis treatment guidelines are based on randomized controlled trials mainly in White individuals. Systemic agents that are commonly used include methotrexate, acitretin, ciclosporin, and apremilast. Genetic polymorphisms in some ethnicities (South Indian Tamils) suggest a superior response to methotrexate than other populations.

Biological treatment with anti-tumor necrosis factor (TNF) (adalimumab, certolizumab, etanercept, infliximab), anti-IL-12/23 (ustekinumab), anti-IL-23 (guselkumab, risankizumab, tildrakizumab), anti-IL-17 (secukinumab, ixekizumab), and anti-IL-17 receptor A (IL-17RA) (brodalumab) have shown efficacy in all racial groups (Figure 3.3). However, in the Phase III REVEAL study, adalimumab showed greater efficacy in White participants than non-White subjects.[11]

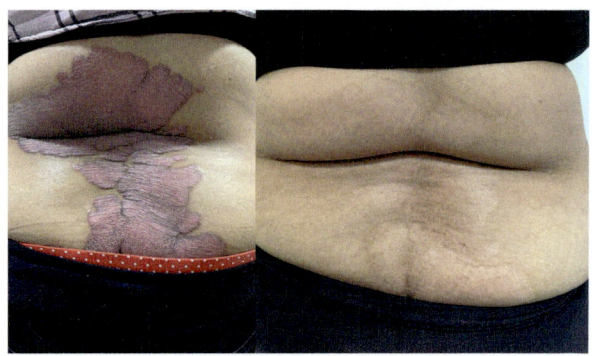

Figure 3.3 Before (left) and after (right) treatment of chronic plaque psoriasis with a biological agent.

3.4 Hidradenitis suppurativa

Hidradenitis suppurativa (HS) has been found to be more prevalent in people with SOC and those of lower socioeconomic status, although the reasons for this are unknown. In the USA, HS has been reported to disproportionately affect female African Americans, while studies in Malaysia have reported a high prevalence in individuals of Indian descent.[12,13] Environmental risk factors include obesity and metabolic syndrome and increased sweating in tropical climates.

Clinical presentation. The clinical course of HS is variable, but initially presents with persistent or recurrent inflammatory lesions, predominantly in single or multiple apocrine gland-bearing areas such as the axillae, groin, and under the breasts (Figure 3.4a). The clinical manifestations are more advanced on presentation in SOC than in white skin. Examination of all body areas in which the condition occurs is essential.

Management. A variety of topical and systemic agents have been used in the management of HS.
Topical treatments tend to have limited efficacy. Topical 1% clindamycin, benzoyl peroxide, and azelaic acid may be helpful in mild HS. Isolated nodules may respond to intralesional triamcinolone injections in combination with oral and topical agents.
Systemic treatment. The most studied antibiotic combination for HS is clindamycin with rifampicin (both 300 mg twice a day) for

12 weeks. Doxycycline, 100 mg/day, is the preferred long-term antibiotic for maintenance.

Given that insulin resistance and hyperandrogenemia may worsen HS, adjuvant therapy with metformin, 0.5–2.5 g/day, may be helpful. Dapsone, 50–200 mg/day, acitretin, ciclosporin, and oral prednisolone have been used in people with SOC. Hormonal therapies such as spironolactone, 50–200 mg/day, and finasteride, 1–5 mg/day, can be considered in patients with co-existing PCOS and obesity. Zinc supplementation of 90 mg/day may also be beneficial.

Biological treatment with TNFα inhibitors (adalimumab) and IL-17 inhibitors (secukinumab) can be considered in patients with severe disease (Figure 3.4b).

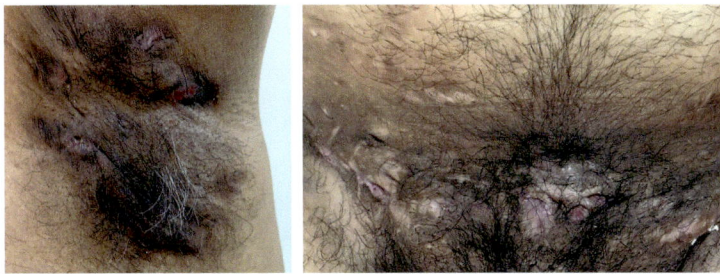

Figure 3.4a Hidradenitis suppurativa: (left) axillary; (right) suprapubic.

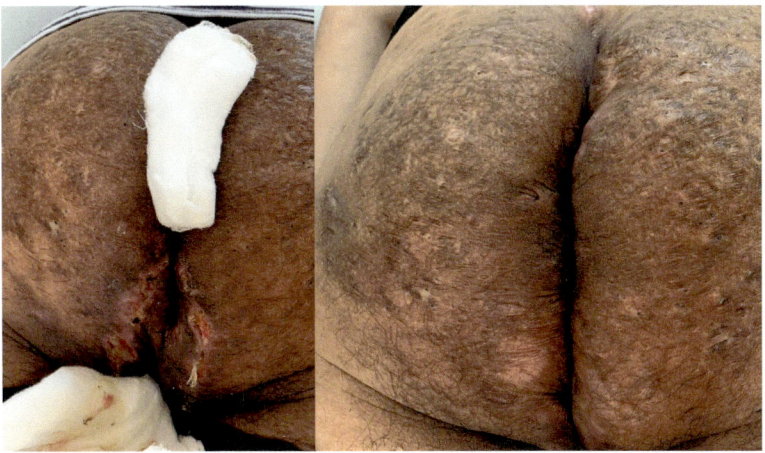

Figure 3.4b Hidradenitis suppurativa before (left) and after (right) treatment with a biological agent (tumor necrosis factor α inhibitor).

Wide local excision is the only curative treatment but may require care by multidisciplinary teams.

3.5 Post-inflammatory hyperpigmentation

PIH is temporary pigmentation that occurs frequently in SOC. It may follow inflammatory dermatoses like acne, eczema, psoriasis, or lichen planus, or may occur because of external triggers such as sunlight exposure, injury, or some medications. PIH can persist for several years and cause considerable emotional distress.[14]

Clinical presentation. PIH manifests as hyperpigmented patches (light brown to black) at the site of the original disease or injury after it has resolved (Figure 3.5). UV radiation can darken the pigmentation further.

Management. In most cases, patients can be reassured that the PIH will resolve with time.

Photoprotection (see pages 85–86) with tinted sunscreens can help prevent PIH to a certain extent and minimize darkening caused by exposure to UV and visible light.

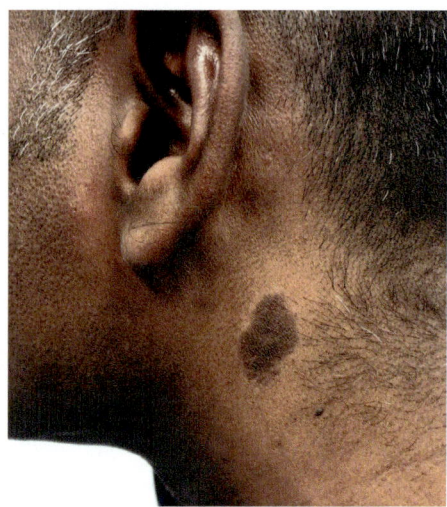

Figure 3.5 Post-inflammatory hyperpigmentation following lichen planus.

Topical treatment. The gold standard treatment for PIH is the combination of hydroquinone, retinoids, and steroids. Hydroquinone (usually 4%) and retinoids can also be used as monotherapy. For acne-related PIH, topical tazarotene (0.045%) and tretinoin (0.05%) may be helpful. Topical thiamidol, azelaic acid, and vitamin C may also be efficacious and do not cause skin irritation.

Physical treatments. Superficial peels with acid concentrations of 20–50% can be used. Deeper peels may cause exacerbation of pigmentary changes in SOC. Glycolic and salicylic acid can be used in combination with the topical agents mentioned above.

Laser treatment with low fluence Q-switched neodymium-doped (Nd):YAG may be beneficial. However, worsening of pigmentation, pain, blistering, and scarring can occur.

Alternative therapies include platelet-rich plasma, oral tranexamic acid (500 mg twice a day), and botanical products such as bakuchiol.

3.6 Skin cancer

In general, there is a lower incidence of skin cancer in individuals with SOC compared with white-skinned people. Deeper skin tones have more melanin, which filters UV light, a major risk factor for the development of skin cancer in White populations. However, people with SOC still develop skin cancer, often in less sun-exposed sites (palms, soles, toe- and fingernails, groin, genitals, and inside the mouth), and mortality rates are disproportionately high in people of color, partly because of diagnostic delays.[15]

Squamous cell carcinoma (SCC) is the most common cutaneous malignancy in Black and Asian Indian people, representing 30–65% of skin cancers in both races.[15,16] SCC occurs on sun-protected sites in Black people, which calls into question UV radiation as an important etiologic factor. Instead, key risk factors for the development of SCC in black skin are chronic scarring processes and chronic inflammation. SCC develops in burn scars, areas of past physical or thermal trauma, sites of previous radiation therapy, and areas of chronic inflammation such as ulcers. SCC that develops within a chronic scarring process tends to be more aggressive and is associated with a 20–40% risk of metastasis.[16]

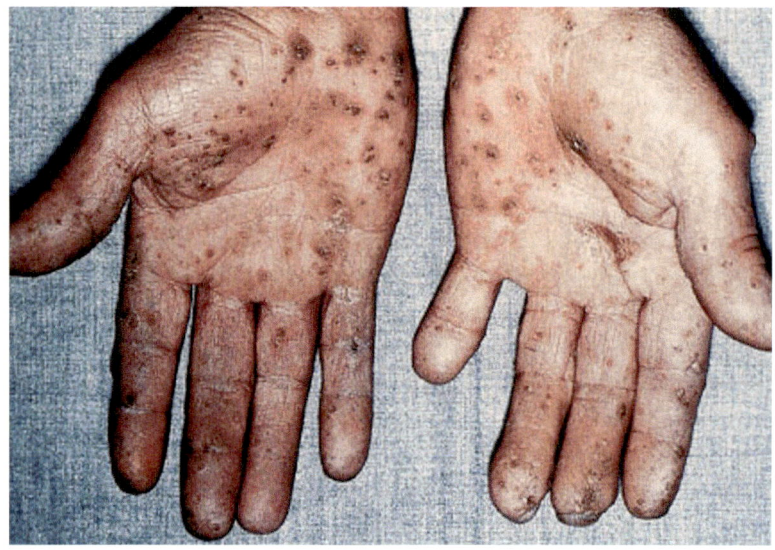

Figure 3.6a Arsenical keratosis of the palms, with multiple Bowen's disease papules and early squamous cell carcinomas.

Clinical presentation. SCCs are often superficial, discrete, hard lesions of variable appearance that arise from an indurated, rounded, and elevated base (Figure 3.6a). They have the potential to metastasize.

Management. Non-healing ulcers should be biopsied, regardless of original etiology, if they have been present for a significant amount of time.

Treatment options for superficial lesions of Bowen's disease (SCC in situ) include cryotherapy, curettage with electrosurgery, surgical excision, and topical 5-fluorouracil or imiquimod. Invasive lesions can be managed with surgical excision, with regular follow-up dependent on the risk factors.

Basal cell carcinoma (BCC) is the second most common cutaneous malignancy in Black and Asian Indian people.[16] It is equally predominant in men and women with SOC, whereas it is more common in White men. BCC is primarily related to intensive UV light exposure and occurs most often in people over 50 years old on sun-exposed areas of the head and neck.

Clinical presentation. BCCs often present as asymptomatic, translucent, solitary nodules with central ulceration. More than 50% of them are pigmented in SOC (Figure 3.6b) compared with only 5% of BCCs in white skin. BCCs in Asian people are brown to glossy black with a so-called 'black pearly' appearance. They may be mistaken for seborrheic keratosis or melanoma. Lesions can occur as nodules, plaques, papules, or ulcers. In more advanced cases, BCCs can present as indurated or pedunculated masses.

Management. A biopsy can be considered, though the clinical features may be sufficient to make a definitive diagnosis. Treatment options include surgical excision, radiotherapy, cryosurgery, curettage with electrosurgery, and topical 5-fluorouracil or imiquimod. Choice of treatment depends on the size, location, and histological subtype of the lesion, as well as the patient's preference, age, and health.

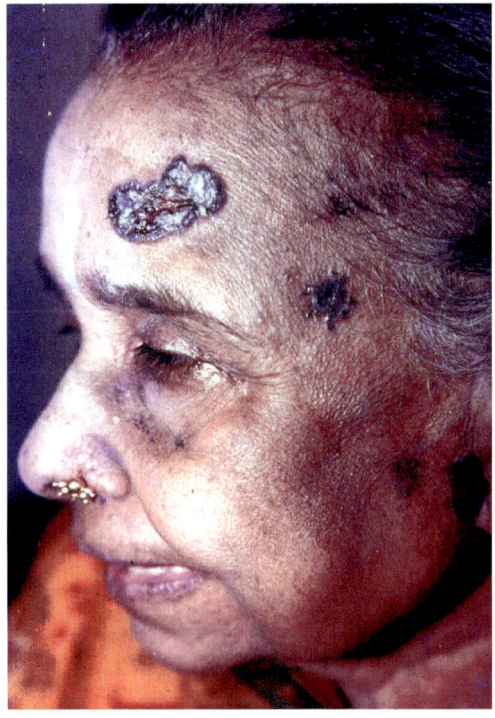

Figure 3.6b Multiple pigmented basal cell carcinomas.

Malignant melanoma has a much lower incidence in SOC than white skin; however, it is often diagnosed at more advanced stages resulting in lower survival rates.[16] Risk factors for melanoma in SOC include burn scars, radiation therapy, trauma, immunosuppression, and pre-existing pigmented lesions (especially on acral and mucosal regions). A family history of melanoma is a significant risk factor in White people but does not appear to be a major predisposing factor in Black people.

Clinical presentation. In contrast to white skin, melanomas most often arise on non-sun-exposed SOC that has less pigment, particularly acral areas of the lower extremities. Mucous membranes and acral areas are the most common sites of melanoma in non-White people, with 60–75% of tumors arising on the palms (Figure 3.6c), soles, mucosal locations, and subungual regions. In 25–50% of cases, malignant melanomas arise within prior pigmented lesions.[16]

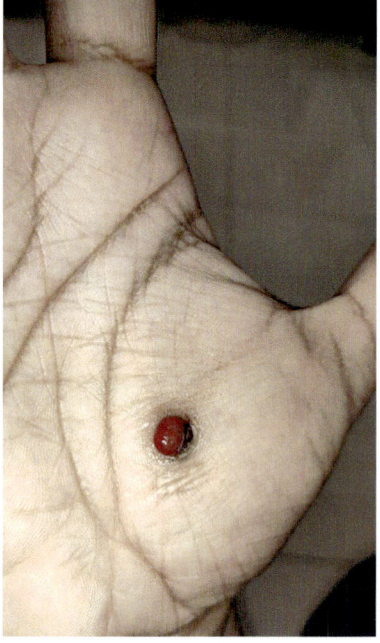

Figure 3.6c Malignant amelanotic melanoma.

The predominant melanoma subtype in SOC is acral lentiginous melanoma on the lower extremities, palms, soles, and nail beds. Hispanic and Black people in the USA usually present with more advanced, thicker melanomas than White people, and tend to have a poorer prognosis with higher mortality. This could be due to delayed diagnosis, as patients are often unaware of the risks of melanoma in dark skin, or due to dermatologists not picking it up early. Melanoma can metastasize widely.

Management. Surgical excision is the definitive treatment for cutaneous melanoma after the diagnosis has been confirmed by excisional biopsy. A portion of normal skin is also removed from around the lesion to prevent local recurrence. As melanoma cells have the capacity to migrate locally from the original tumor, sentinel lymph node biopsy may be required for melanomas beyond a certain thickness histologically.

Self-examination. Patients should be educated about the risk of developing skin cancer and how to perform a monthly self-examination of their skin in front of a full-length mirror. A handheld mirror is also useful for checking hard-to-see areas. Patients should seek medical attention if they find any new or changing lesion or anything unusual. Sun damage in SOC presents as uneven skin tone, PIH, melasma, or a combination of these characteristics rather than lines and wrinkles. Dark lines under or around the fingernails or toenails and sores that won't heal are further red flags for medical attention.

Photoprotection. Although SOC has more melanin in the epidermis and repairs DNA damage more efficiently than white skin, it is still at significant risk of damage from UV radiation. Patients should be advised to take measures to protect the skin from sun damage (Table 3.1). Studies have shown that daily photoprotection in SOC helps to prevent the development of skin cancer, avoid photoaging such as uneven skin tone, and prevent exacerbating pigmentary disorders such as melasma and PIH.[17,18]

Broad-spectrum sunscreens with sun protection factor (SPF) 30 or higher are recommended. However, these do not protect against visible light and long-wave UVA, which contributes to disorders of

TABLE 3.1

Photoprotection measures

- Seek shade when outdoors
- Wear photoprotective clothing
  - Wide-brimmed hat
  - Fabrics with a tight weave, dark color, and heavy weight
- Apply broad-spectrum, water-resistant, tinted sunscreens (SPF 30 or greater)
- Reapply sunscreen at regular intervals
- Never use tanning beds or sunlamps

SPF, sun protection factor.

hyperpigmentation. Sunscreens containing zinc oxide, titanium dioxide, and iron oxides provide protection against a broad range of wavelengths including visible light but may leave a whitish residue on the skin. Formulas containing ultralight textures, sprays, non-greasy formulations, and tinted sunscreens are excellent alternatives. Tinted sunscreens combine a colored base with UV filters and camouflage uneven skin tone (Figure 3.6d).[17]

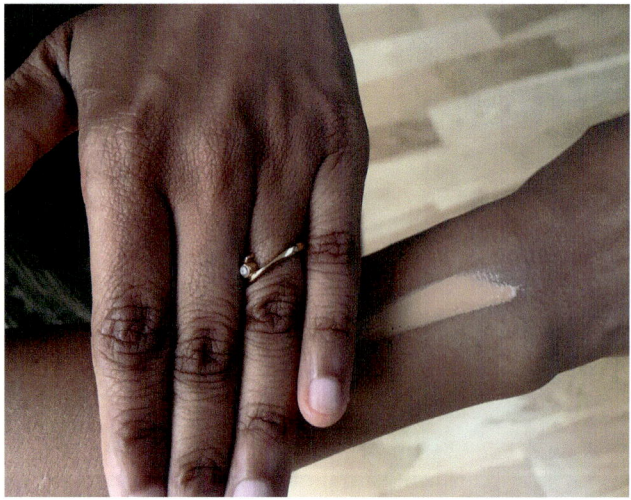

Figure 3.6d Tinted sunscreen applied to skin of color.

Supplemental oral antioxidants, including vitamin E, vitamin C, and carotenoids may be beneficial.

3.7 Psychological factors

A variety of skin conditions can cause significant psychosocial distress, particularly in individuals with SOC. In a recent US survey, nearly 80% of 501 respondents with SOC reported a moderate-to-severe skin condition, with 57% saying that their condition affected their mental health.[19]

Pigmentary disorders, such as melasma, PIH, and vitiligo, are among the top dermatological concerns for people with SOC (Figure 3.7a). Even mild forms of facial pigmentation can be detrimental to quality of life, particularly for women. Validated, easy-to-use psychiatric screening tools can be used to detect psychological problems in patients with pigmentary disorders, so that appropriate support and counseling can be provided.

Melasma, which causes hyperpigmentation on the face and other sun-exposed areas (Figure 3.7b), can be associated with profound psychosocial effects. Studies have indicated that melasma is more prevalent in people with SOC, particularly in women because it can be triggered by hormones during pregnancy and hormonal medications.

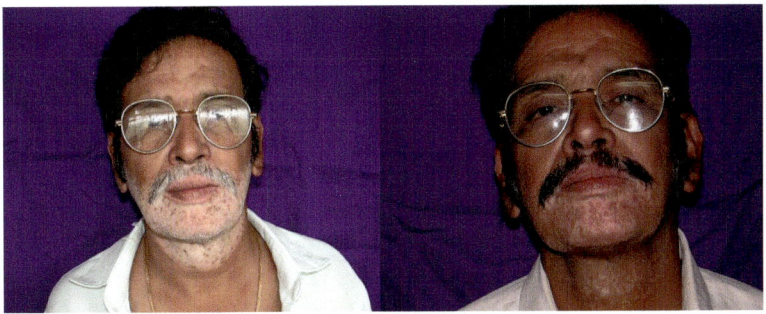

Figure 3.7a Depigmentation after use of hair dye (left) and repigmentation after avoidance of dye (right).

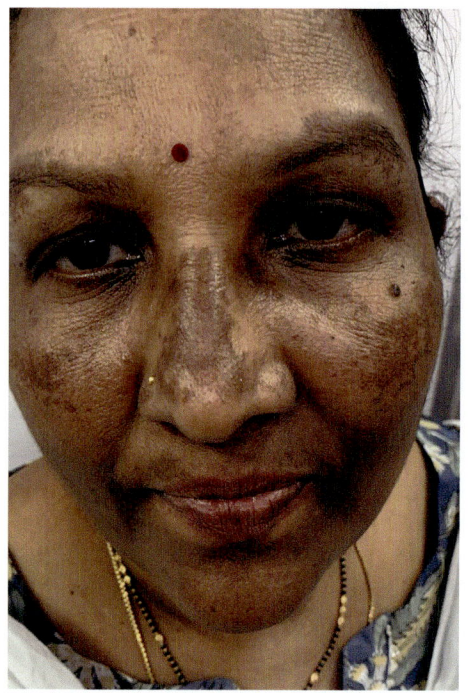

Figure 3.7b Melasma.

Internalized stigma or the acceptance of negative societal stereotypes are primary factors for the psychological burden. One study in India found that 11.6% of 86 patients with melasma had anxiety, 12.8% had depression, and 8.1% had somatoform disorder.[20]

Vitiligo is often mistaken for leprosy on the Indian subcontinent, which causes significant distress to those who develop it and impairs quality of life. In the Indian study, 21% of 95 patients with vitiligo had anxiety, 27% had depression, and 17.9% had somatoform disorder.[20] The stigma of vitiligo may limit the chances of marriage in young women who manifest patches in visible areas (Figure 3.7c). Older patients or those who develop the disease later in life adjust better to this chronic dermatosis.

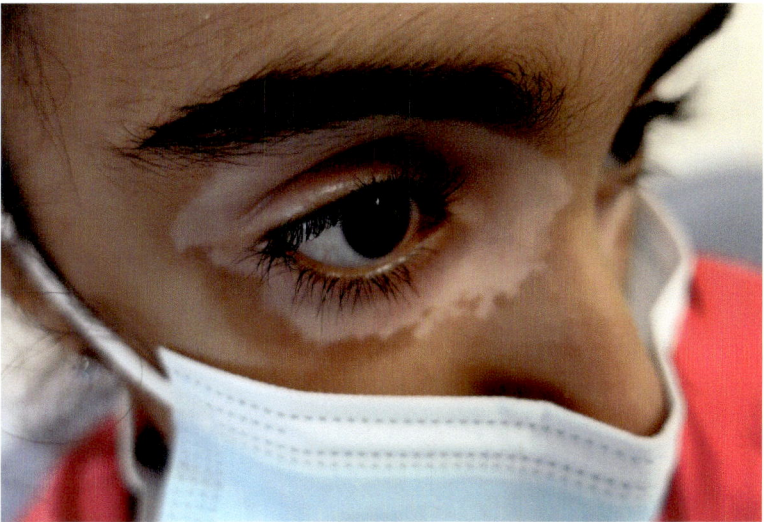

Figure 3.7c Vitiligo.

Hidradenitis suppurativa has an increased prevalence, and tends to be more severe, in individuals with SOC than those with white skin (see pages 78–80). It has been shown to cause significant embarrassment and social isolation, affect intimate relationships and sexual activity, cause anxiety and depression, and reduce quality of life. Large population studies are needed to better understand the prevalence and burden of HS in patients with SOC. When diagnosing and treating the condition, healthcare providers need to be aware that psychological support may also be required.[21]

Psoriasis is associated with greater psychological impact, lower quality of life, and higher scores on the Dermatology Life Quality Index in people with SOC than those with white skin (see page 77). This may be due to post-inflammatory pigmentary sequelae and cultural variations in perceptions of skin disorders with associated negative effects. In a study undertaken by the National Psoriasis Foundation, 72% of minorities reported that psoriasis had an impact on their quality of life (compared with 54% of Caucasian respondents). Specific problems included self-consciousness, embarrassment, anger, frustration, and helplessness.[9]

Key points – presentation and management of common dermatoses in skin of color

- Acne, eczema, and psoriasis are more common, and often more severe, in people with SOC than those with white skin.
- PIH is a common sequela of dermatoses such as acne, eczema, and psoriasis. It is usually temporary but can cause significant emotional distress.
- SOC presents with common dermatoses in different ways from lighter skin tones. For example, erythema may present as shades of violet or an increase in pigmentation rather than redness as seen in white skin.
- There is limited evidence of effectiveness of treatments for common dermatoses in people with SOC because they tend to be under-represented in clinical trials.
- Although there is a lower incidence of skin cancer in SOC than white skin, it is often diagnosed at a more advanced stage in less sun-exposed areas of the body, resulting in a disproportionately high rate of mortality.
- Patients with SOC should be educated with regards to photoprotection measures to avoid sun damage and prevent exacerbations of pigmentary disorders.
- The need for psychological support must be considered as part of the management plan for common dermatoses in people with SOC, who may experience social stigma, anxiety, and depression because of their condition.

References

1. Perkins AC, Cheng CE, Hillebrand GG, et al. Comparison of the epidemiology of acne vulgaris among Caucasian, Asian, Continental Indian and African American women. *J Eur Acad Dermatol Venereol.* 2011;25(9):1054-1060.
2. Kim JJ, Choi YM. Phenotype and genotype of polycystic ovary syndrome in Asia: ethnic differences. *J Obstet Gynaecol Res.* 2019;45(12):2330-2337.
3. Eichenfield DZ, Sprague J, Eichenfield LF. Management of acne vulgaris: a review. *JAMA.* 2021;326(20):2055-2067.

4. Chiang C, Ward M, Gooderham M. Dermatology: how to manage acne in skin of colour. *Drugs Context.* 2022;11:2021-10-19.
5. Havelin A, Seukeran DC. Laser treatment of acne scarring in skin of colour. *Clin Exp Dermatol.* 2023;48(5):443-447.
6. Sachdeva M, Joseph M. Dermatology: how to manage atopic dermatitis in patients with skin of colour. *Drugs Context.* 2022;11:2021-12-1.
7. Gan C, Mahil S, Pink A, Rodrigues M. Atopic dermatitis in skin of colour. Part 2: considerations in clinical presentation and treatment options. *Clin Exp Dermatol.* 2023;48(10):1091-1101.
8. Stein CM, Sadeque A, Murray JJ, Wandel C. Cyclosporine pharmacokinetics and pharmacodynamics in African American and white subjects. *Clin Pharmacol Ther.* 2001;69(5):317-323.
9. Alexis AF, Blackcloud P. Psoriasis in skin of color: epidemiology, genetics, clinical presentation, and treatment nuances. *J Clin Aesthet Dermatol.* 2014;7(11):16-24.
10. Kim J, Oh CH, Jeon J, et al. Molecular phenotyping small (Asian) versus large (Western) plaque psoriasis shows common activation of IL-17 pathway genes but different regulatory gene sets. *J Invest Dermatol.* 2016;136(1):161-172.
11. Menter A, Gordon KB, Leonardi CL, Gu Y, Goldblum OM. Efficacy and safety of adalimumab across subgroups of patients with moderate to severe type psoriasis. *J Am Acad Dermatol.* 2010;63(3):448-456.
12. Zouboulis CC, Goyal M, Byrd AS. Hidradenitis suppurativa in skin of color. *Exp Dermatol.* 2021;30(Suppl 1):27-30.
13. Choi ECE, Phan PHC, Oon HH. Hidradenitis suppurativa: racial and socioeconomic considerations in management. *Int J Dermatol.* 2022;61(12):1452-1457.
14. Anvery N, Christensen RE, Dirr MA. Management of post-inflammatory hyperpigmentation in skin of color. *J Cosmet Dermatol.* 2022;21:1837-1840.
15. Gupta AK, Bharadwaj M, Mehrotra R. Skin cancer concerns in people of color: risk factors and prevention. *Asian Pac J Cancer Prev.* 2016;17(12):5257-5264.
16. Gloster HM, Neal K. Skin cancer in skin of color. *J Am Acad Dermatol.* 2006;55(5):741-760; quiz 761-764.
17. Krutmann J, Piquero-Casals J, Morgado-Carrasco D, et al. Photoprotection for people with skin of colour: needs and strategies. *Br J Dermatol.* 2023;188(2):168-175.

18. Taylor SC, Alexis AF, Armstrong AW, Chiesa Fuxench ZC, Lim HW. Misconceptions of photoprotection in skin of color. *J Am Acad Dermatol.* 2022;86:S9-S17.
19. Cartwright MM, Kamen T, Desai SR. The psychosocial burden of skin disease and dermatology care insights among skin of color consumers. *J Drugs Dermatol.* 2023;22(10):1027-1033.
20. Dabas G, Vinay K, Parsad D, Kumar A, Kumaran MS. Psychological disturbances in patients with pigmentary disorders: a cross-sectional study. *J Eur Acad Dermatol Venereol.* 2020;34(2):392-399.
21. Lee DE, Clark AK, Shi VY. Hidradenitis suppurativa: disease burden and etiology in skin of color. *Dermatology.* 2017;233(6):456-461.

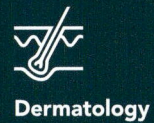

4 Presentation and management of dermatoses predominantly seen in skin of color

4.1 Mycosis fungoides *94*
4.2 Dermal melanocytosis (Mongolian blue spot) *95*
4.3 Kumkum/bindi-induced dermatitis *96*
4.4 Dermatosis papulosa nigra *97*
4.5 Dermatitis cruris pustulosa et atrophicans *98*
4.6 Parthenium dermatitis *99*
4.7 Cydnidae pigmentation *101*
4.8 Pseudofolliculitis barbae *102*
4.9 Macular amyloidosis *103*
4.10 Lichen planus pigmentosus *104*
4.11 Actinic lichen planus *106*
4.12 Maturational hyperpigmentation *107*
4.13 Disseminated infundibulofolliculitis *109*
4.14 Arsenical keratosis *110*
4.15 Exogenous ochronosis *111*
4.16 Confluent and reticulate papillomatosis *112*
4.17 Tinea versicolor *113*
4.18 Keloids *114*
4.19 Post-kala-azar dermal leishmaniasis *115*
4.20 Physiological melanonychia striata *116*
4.21 Creeping eruptions in the skin *118*

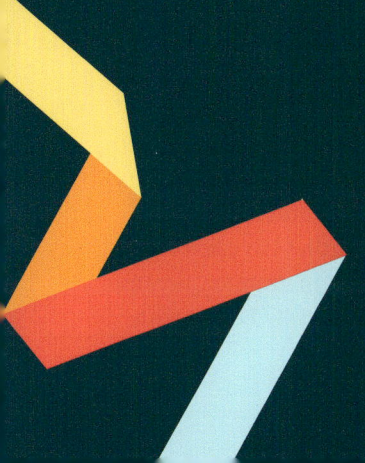

HEALTHCARE

The dermatoses discussed in this chapter are unique to, or more prevalent in, people with skin of color (SOC).

4.1 Mycosis fungoides

The incidence of mycosis fungoides (MF), a form of cutaneous T-cell lymphoma (CTCL), is higher among Black than White people and other racial groups, but this difference decreases with age.[1] CTCL also follows a more aggressive course in Black people than White people, with a higher mortality rate. Studies have shown that early-stage MF is more likely to go undetected or be misdiagnosed in black skin compared with lighter skin tones; prompt recognition of MF in SOC may improve outcomes.[2]

Clinical presentation. There are three common, often intertwined, presentations of classic MF in SOC. First, the asymptomatic dyspigmentation associated with MF can manifest as hypo- or hyperpigmentation. The next presentation involves pruritus, secondary lichenification, and hyperpigmentation that often masks clues to the presence of MF. Thirdly, some patients may present with morphologies that mimic more common dermatoses, such as psoriasis, atopic dermatitis, vitiligo, or lichen planus (LP).

The classic morphology is arcuate lesions with scaly, poikilodermatous patches and plaques with atrophy (Figure 4.1). MF lesions are usually a minimum of 5 cm in size. Many of the histological mimics are smaller. The polymorphic pigmentation of MF in SOC usually presents as discrete lesions exhibiting hypopigmentation admixed with hyperpigmentation. Features that are considered 'consistent with' but not classic for MF are erythema, scaly patches and plaques, alopecia, hypopigmentation, hyperpigmentation, and erythroderma.[3] The morphology and distribution of lesions can help in the diagnosis of MF.

Management of MF is similar to that in white skin. Topical steroids, phototherapy, and methotrexate are used according to the severity. Hypopigmented MF may respond better to phototherapy, as ultraviolet (UV) light penetrates affected areas that have less color. In addition, hypopigmented variants are easier to monitor, because pigment returns with remission and relapse typically begins with

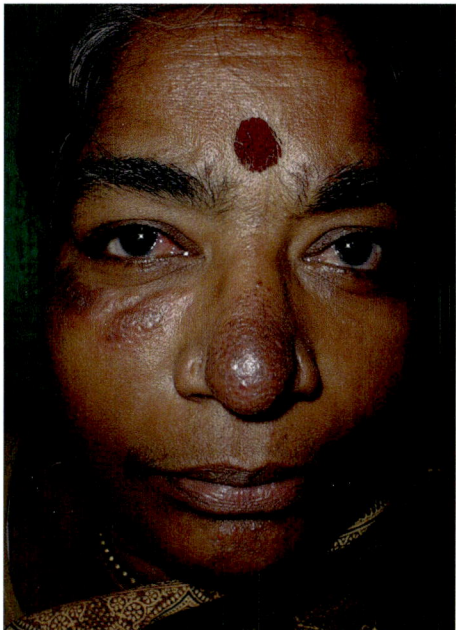

Figure 4.1 Tumid papules and plaques of mycosis fungoides.

hypopigmentation. Conversely, while treatment of hyperpigmented lesions will often eliminate scale and induration, biopsies may be needed to confirm clearance of the disease.

4.2 Dermal melanocytosis (Mongolian blue spot)

Dermal melanocytosis is a relatively common condition seen in children with SOC. It is usually present at birth.[4,5]

Clinical presentation. Dermal melanocytosis usually presents at birth as a single smooth bluish patch, 1–12 cm in size, on normal textured skin (Figure 4.2). Occasionally, children have multiple patches. It usually occurs in the lower sacral region. The blue color fades into the surrounding skin and has no sharp border. Dermal melanocytosis usually disappears at 3–4 years of age, rarely persisting throughout life. It has no systemic significance, but GM1 gangliosidosis type 1 and trisomy 20 mosaicism should be excluded in children with extensive patches.

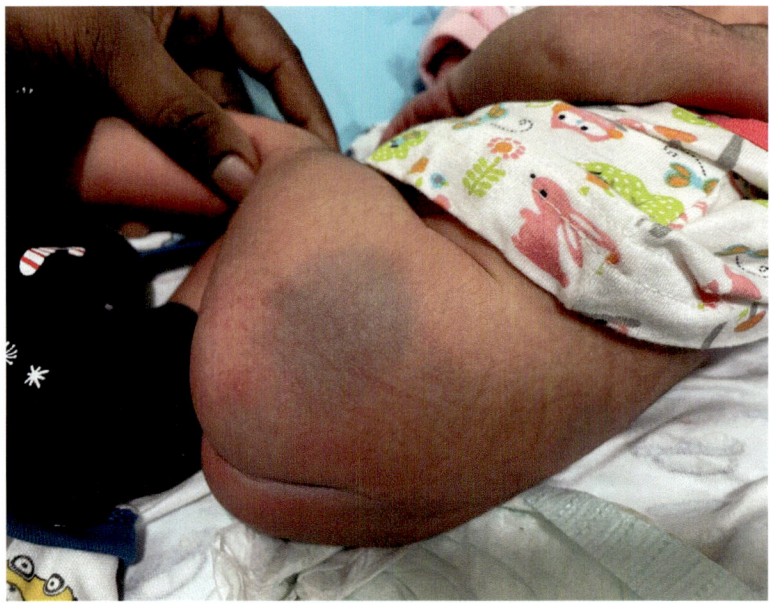

Figure 4.2 Dermal melanocytosis, also known as Mongolian blue spot.

Histopathology shows widely scattered melanin containing melanocytes in the lower half of the dermis. The cells are elongated. Rarely, melanophages may be present.

Management. Parents usually only need reassurance that the condition will resolve with time. In persistent cases, Q-switched neodymium-doped:yttrium-aluminum-garnett (Nd:YAG) laser therapy can provide effective cosmetic results.

4.3 Kumkum/bindi-induced dermatitis

Kumkum, also known as bindi or tilakam, is a mark worn on the center of the forehead by Hindu women. It is deemed compulsory for married women for socioreligious reasons.[6] Kumkum can be prepared at home by mixing turmeric powder with lime juice and alum, and commercial formulations of kumkum are also available, many of which contain azo dyes. More recently, colored discs with adhesive backs that can be stuck to the forehead have become available.

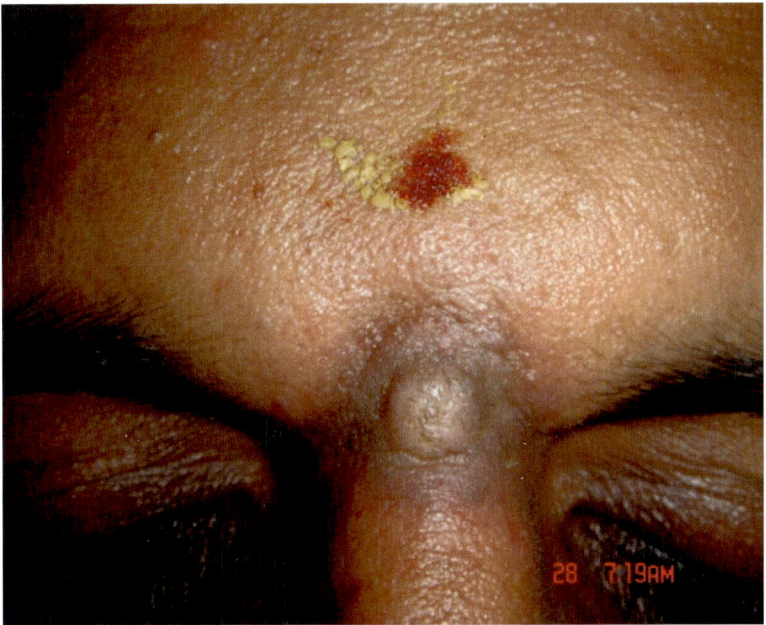

Figure 4.3 Kumkum contact dermatitis.

Clinical presentation. Three types of skin lesions are possible: contact dermatitis (Figure 4.3), hyperpigmentation with or without previous dermatitis, and depigmentation. The last is more predominant in women who use the plastic bindis.

Management. Treatment is difficult since most of the affected women are unwilling to give up the kumkum for socioreligious reasons. However, women with suspected dermatitis should be patch tested and alternative non-allergic materials recommended.

4.4 Dermatosis papulosa nigra
Dermatosis papulosa nigra predominantly affects Black adults, with a highly variable incidence of 10–70%.[7] There is often a family history of this common condition.

Clinical presentation. Dermatosis papulosa nigra presents as multiple, small, hyperpigmented, pedunculated or verrucous papules on the

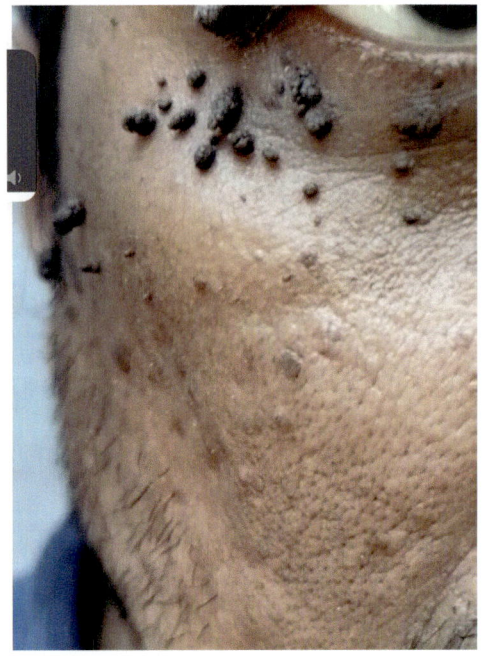

Figure 4.4 Dermatosis papulosa nigra.

malar areas of the face (Figure 4.4) as well as the neck, chest, and back. It starts after puberty, with the papules gradually increasing in number. There is no malignant potential.

Histopathology resembles that of seborrheic keratosis.

Management. The condition is mostly treated for cosmetic reasons. Electrofulguration after a topical anesthetic gives satisfactory results.

4.5 Dermatitis cruris pustulosa et atrophicans

Dermatitis cruris pustulosa et atrophicans (DCPA) is a marvelously mnemonic term given to a chronic folliculitis of the legs found exclusively in people of color.[8]

Clinical presentation. DCPA presents as superficial follicular pustules on the anterior surface of the legs of young men (Figure 4.5),

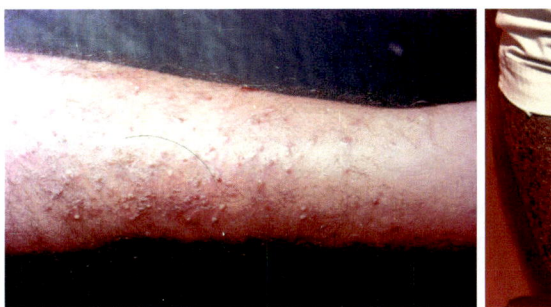
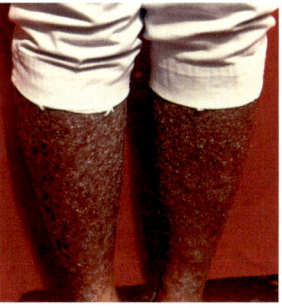

Figure 4.5 Dermatitis cruris pustulosa et atrophicans.

sometimes extending to the thighs. It is occasionally reported in young women, especially those with hairy legs. The pustules persist for a long time. Even if they subside with therapy, they tend to recur soon after treatment is stopped. The interfollicular skin may show eczematous changes and patients may complain of itching. There are no systemic features, and the condition is not painful. After many years of recurrent pustules the skin becomes shiny and atrophic, the hairs are shed, and spontaneous cure occurs.

Investigations. Culture from the pustules regularly grows *Staphylococcus aureus*. Histopathology in the early stages shows many neutrophils around the infundibulum of the hair follicles. As the condition becomes chronic, a lymphocytic infiltrate is seen around the deeper parts of the hair follicle. There are no inflammatory cells in the late atrophic stage, and hair follicles and appendages disappear.

Management. The pustules respond to antibiotics but tend to recur as soon as the drug is stopped even when combinations of antibiotics are used. Topical steroid creams relieve the itching. Anecdotal reports suggest remission with psoralen and ultraviolet A (PUVA), minocycline, and dapsone therapy.

4.6 Parthenium dermatitis

Parthenium hysterophorus, a plant in the Asteraceae family, is a widespread weed in most parts of India. Two major allergens – parthenin and ambrosin – are carried in small organelles on the leaf surface called trichomes. These allergens cause dermatitis, mostly among 40–50-year-old men working in agriculture.⁹

Clinical presentation. Parthenium dermatitis usually starts on the feet and legs of those who work bare footed. The face is often involved due to airborne allergens from the plant (Figure 4.6). The primary lesions are papules and papulo-vesicles. After an initial acute phase, it becomes a chronic condition with marked lichenification and intense pruritus. Though the dermatitis is widespread, the worst affected areas are the exposed sites.

The differential diagnosis includes airborne contact dermatitis, atopic eczema, and seborrheic eczema.

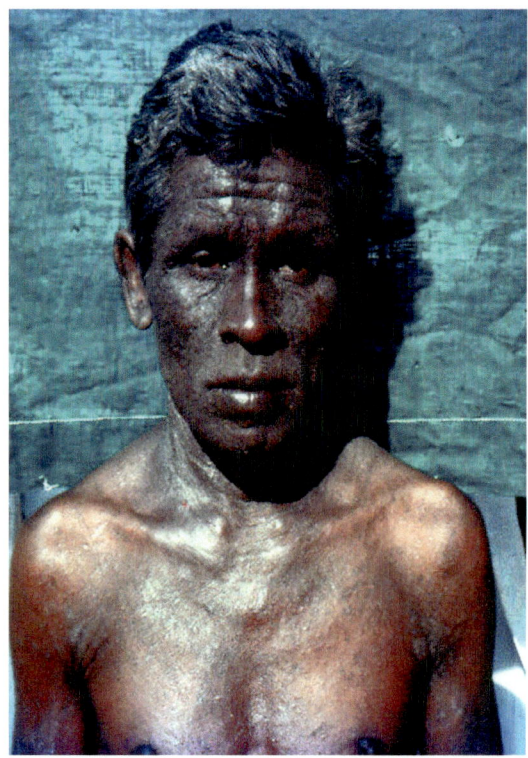

Figure 4.6 Parthenium dermatitis.

Management. Topical and systemic steroids may provide temporary respite. Azathioprine, ciclosporin, and methotrexate can be used as steroid-sparing drugs.

4.7 Cydnidae pigmentation

Cydnidae (burrowing bugs) are arthropods of the order Hemiptera and superfamily Pentatomoidea. They are found in soil and tend to proliferate in warm climates during the rainy season. Cydnidae secrete a substance with a distinctive odor from a gland in the thorax. It is used for self-defense and can cause paralysis in prey.[10]

Clinical presentation. When the secretion comes into contact with human skin it can cause pigmented macules. Most cases report pigmentation on acral sites (Figure 4.7), although pigmentation over the trunk has also been described. The pigmentation has been reproduced in a clinic setting by rubbing the secretion between the thumb and forefinger. It can be difficult to remove the pigment with soap and water during initial assessment. However, it can be rubbed away, with some effort, using acetone.

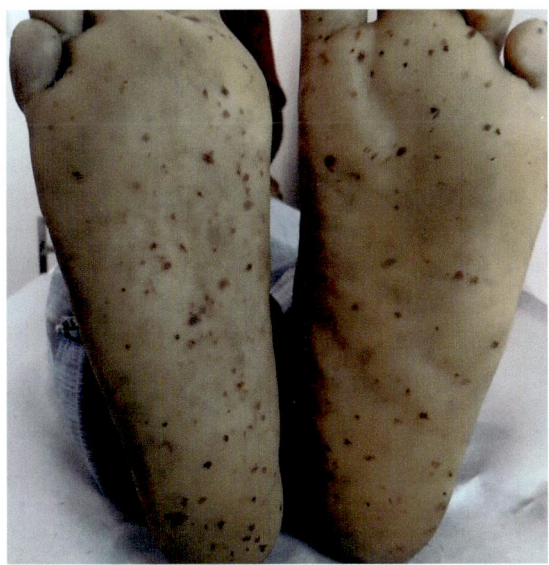

Figure 4.7 Cydnidae pigmentation.

Dermoscopy reveals a cluster of oval to bizarre-shaped brown and shiny globules and clods with a superficial 'stuck-on' appearance. This can be helpful in distinguishing the condition from other differentials for sudden-onset pigmentation in the soles, including septic emboli, contact dermatitis, and eruptive lentigines. Cydnidae pigmentation can be mistaken for the petechiae associated with dengue, which also occurs most commonly during the monsoon season.

Management. The pigment gradually resolves after 6 days when left untreated.

4.8 Pseudofolliculitis barbae

Pseudofolliculitis barbae (PFB) is an inflammatory dermatosis of follicular and perifollicular skin caused by ingrown hairs. A poor shaving technique or other forms of epilation, such as plucking, can leave cut hairs that curl in on themselves, resulting in an inflammatory reaction that emerges a few millimeters away from the sharp-growing hair tips. This is referred to as extrafollicular penetration or transfollicular penetration when it occurs through the follicular wall. Genetic factors play a part in the condition, as the curved shape of African hair predisposes to it.[11]

Clinical presentation. PFB manifests as itchy papules, pustules, and post-inflammatory pigmentation, most commonly in the beard area (Figure 4.8). Patients experience pruritus and pain in the shaved area 1 or 2 days after shaving. Although the pustules are usually sterile, secondary infections may develop. Keloids may also develop in predisposed individuals. PFB can affect self-esteem and quality of life.

Management. Shaving should be stopped at the first sign of active inflammation. Trapped hairs can be removed with a sterile needle. Topical clindamycin, keratolytics, and benzoyl peroxide may reduce moderate inflammatory changes and reduce secondary infection. For more severe inflammation, low-dose tetracyclines, macrolides, or penicillin can be considered. Topical and intralesional steroids may also be beneficial.

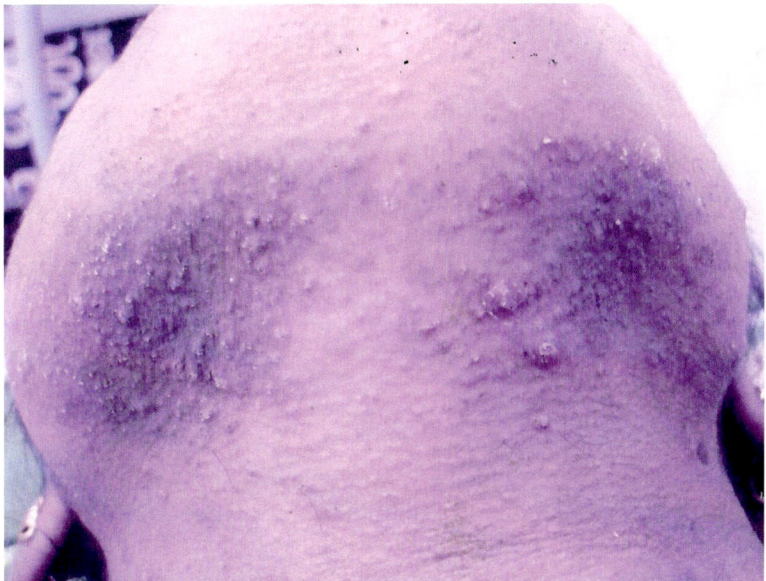

Figure 4.8 Pseudofolliculitis barbae due to plucking of hair in the beard area.

Altering the shaving technique is also essential. Patients should be advised to use electric clippers set at a minimum of 1 mm and to avoid pulling or stretching the skin while shaving with a razor. Dry shaving and shaving against the grain should also be discouraged.

4.9 Macular amyloidosis

Macular amyloidosis is a form of localized cutaneous amyloidosis. Lichen amyloidosis and macular amyloidosis are clinical variants of the same process. The condition is common in Asia, the Middle East, and South America.[12]

Clinical presentation. Macular amyloidosis presents as poorly defined pigmented patches. It has a rippled appearance with parallel bands or ridges of pigmentation, usually on the trunk (Figure 4.9). The rippled pattern is best appreciated by stretching the skin. It has a predilection for the interscapular region. It may be pruritic, but most patients are concerned about the cosmetic appearance.

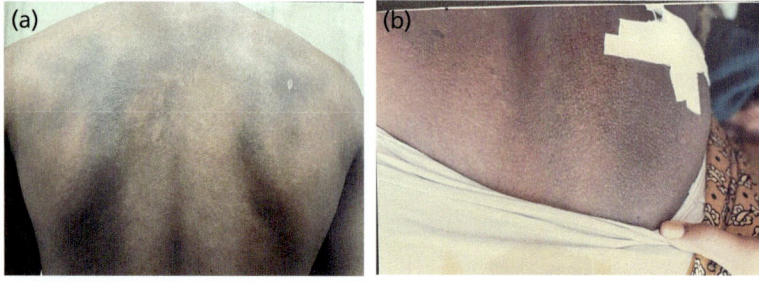

Figure 4.9 (a) Ill-defined pigmented patches on the upper back. (b) Rippled pigmentation of amyloid.

In Japan, cases were reported following prolonged rubbing of the affected area with nylon brushes. In India, the friction caused by vigorous rubbing of the back after a bath using the religious thread worn by some men of the Brahmin community was reported to cause the condition.

Histopathology shows small globular deposits of amyloid in the papillary dermis. Though demonstrable even with the standard hematoxylin-eosin stain, it is best seen with crystal violet on Congo Red stains.

Management. Topical application of corticosteroid or tacrolimus relieves the itching and reduces the pigmentation. Q-switched Nd:YAG laser therapy can improve the cosmetic appearance.

4.10 Lichen planus pigmentosus

Lichen planus pigmentosus (LPP) is a variant of LP that is more common in Asian Indians but has also been reported among other racial and ethnic populations. Provoking factors include sun exposure and the use of mustard and amla oil for body massage. Mustard oil contains allyl isothiocyanate, which is a strong photosensitizer. Long-term use of hair dyes that contain paraphenylenediamine (PPD) can also cause pigmented cosmetic dermatitis. Gradual hyperpigmentation occurs without preceding erythema or itching.[13]

Clinical presentation. LPP has an insidious onset, appearing as dark brown macules on sun-exposed skin and in skin folds, without pruritus. The face and neck are usually involved, particularly the preauricular area (Figure 4.10). The pigmentation subsequently spreads to involve the upper limbs, back, and trunk. LPP has a chronic course, with classic LP lesions occurring in 25% of patients.

Histopathology shows a lichenoid reaction similar to LP. There is damage to the basal layer with pigment incontinence. Melanophages may be present in the upper dermis. The various hues in different patients depend on the 'Tyndal effect' and the baseline complexion of the patient.

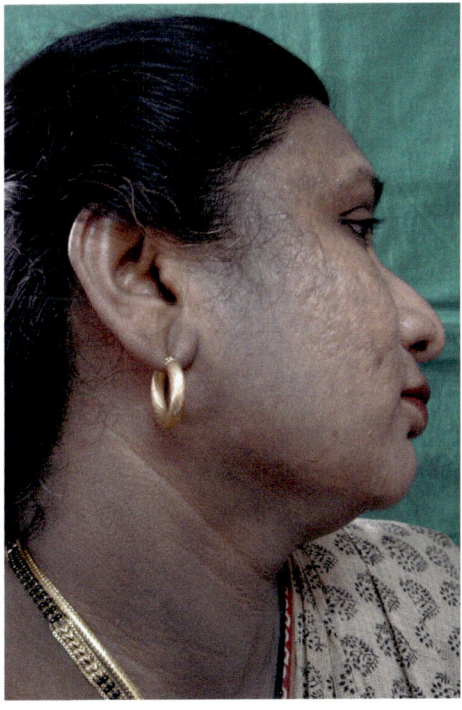

Figure 4.10 Lichen planus pigmentosus.

Differential diagnoses include erythema dyschromicum perstans, Riehl melanosis, idiopathic eruptive macular pigmentation, and pigmented cosmetic dermatitis. There is considerable overlap between these conditions, but they can all be categorized as acquired dermal macular hyperpigmentation as suggested in the Delphi consensus.[14]

Management. There is no established treatment for LPP. Topical treatment with steroid creams and tacrolimus may help. Oral corticosteroids, large doses of vitamin A, and oral synthetic retinoids have anecdotally been described as effective. In select cases, Q-switched Nd:YAG laser therapy has been shown to improve the cosmetic appearance.

4.11 Actinic lichen planus

Actinic lichen planus (ALP), also called lichen planus subtropicus or lichen planus actinicus, affects sun-exposed areas of the skin and is more common in people with SOC than those with white skin. The condition tends to flare in spring and summer, with relative quiescence during the winter months.[15]

Clinical presentation. ALP can present in three forms: annular, pigmented, and dyschromic. Annular ALP manifests as erythematous or brownish annular plaques with or without atrophy (Figure 4.11). Pigmented ALP resembles melasma (see pages 87–88). Dyschromic ALP is rare and presents with whitish, pinhead, and coalescing papules. The face and extensor upper limbs are the most affected sites. Mucosal involvement and Koebnerization are usually absent in this variant.
  Histopathology reveals features of classic LP.

Management. ALP is first treated with topical steroids and calcineurin inhibitors to switch off the inflammatory changes. Some patients may also require oral steroids, hydroxychloroquine, or retinoids. Pigmentation can then be reduced with good photoprotective measures, laser therapy (intense pulsed light), and oral tranexamic acid.

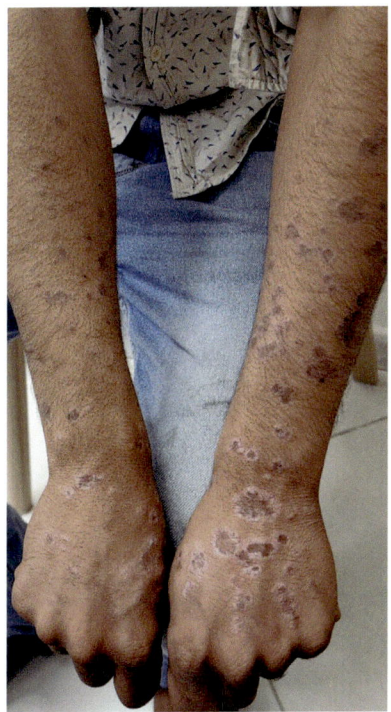

Figure 4.11 Actinic lichen planus.

4.12 Maturational hyperpigmentation

Maturational hyperpigmentation is an acquired facial hypermelanosis that occurs on both cheeks (Figure 4.12). Most cases are observed in individuals of African or Indian descent.[16]

Clinical presentation. Unlike melasma, which has distinct margins and an expansive distribution, maturational hyperpigmentation is usually ill defined and is limited to part of the cheek only. The condition is usually asymptomatic, and patients present to dermatologists with cosmetic concerns.

Fasting hyperglycemia and hyperinsulinemia are observed in more than 70% of patients with maturational hyperpigmentation, so it is a potential cutaneous marker of metabolic syndrome, particularly diabetes.[17]

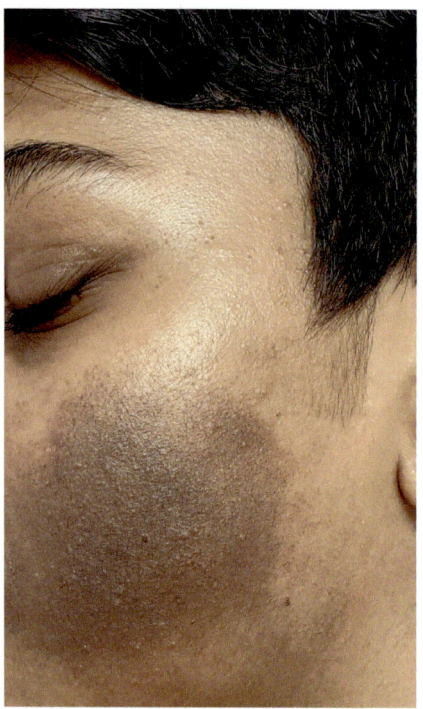

Figure 4.12 Maturational hyperpigmentation.

Histopathology. Biopsy shows melanocyte proliferation in the basal cell layer of the epidermis. Features of post-inflammatory hyperpigmentation (PIH) are absent.

Differential diagnoses include melasma, exogenous ochronosis, LPP, PIH, friction melanosis, and facial acanthosis nigricans. However, maturational hyperpigmentation has fairly specific features, including a relatively soft surface with conspicuous but fine granularity and indistinct margins on gross morphology, as well as suggestive changes on dermoscopy and histopathology.

Management. In addition to lifestyle changes, specific treatments include topical agents like retinoids, hydroquinone, and salicylic acid, chemical peels, and laser therapy.

4.13 Disseminated infundibulofolliculitis

Disseminated infundibulofolliculitis is a condition of unknown etiology that predominantly occurs in people of color. Patients usually present for cosmetic reasons.[18]

Clinical presentation. The condition manifests as a recurrent follicular eruption, mainly on the trunk (Figure 4.13). It is asymptomatic but may itch during the summer months. The papules are skin colored and appear in crops, with a few pustules in between. Each crop may last from several weeks to months.

Histopathology reveals spongiosis and mononuclear cell infiltrate, mainly at the level of the infundibulum of the hair.

Management. Topical steroids can be used to alleviate the itching. Oral isotretinoin may also help.

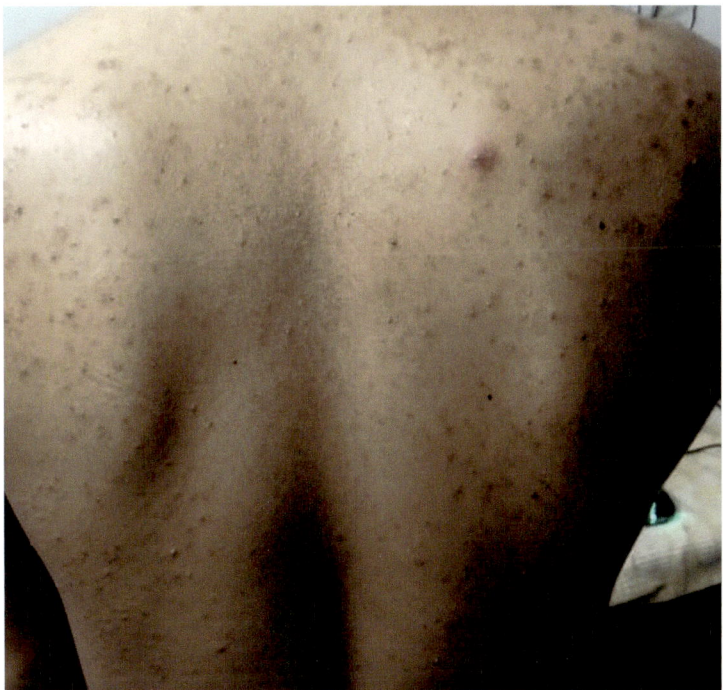

Figure 4.13 Disseminated infundibulofolliculitis.

4.14 Arsenical keratosis

Arsenic is known as the king of poisons and the poison of kings. It has also been used in the past therapeutically as Fowler's solution in the West. Arsenic is also sometimes used as an alternative medicine in India and China. In some parts of the world where the well water is contaminated with high levels of arsenic the metal may get into the food cycle, resulting in chronic arsenic intoxication.[19]

Clinical presentation. The skin provides useful clues to the existence of chronic arsenic poisoning, with the development of pre-cancerous keratotic papules on the palms and soles (Figure 4.14). In the early stages, these papules are more easily felt than seen.

Over time, some of the keratotic papules may turn into Bowen's disease, basal cell carcinoma, or squamous cell carcinoma (see Chapter 3). The period before malignant transformation is unpredictable and may be as long as 40 years.

Diffuse pigmentation interspersed with macular areas of depigmentation is sometimes described as 'rain drops on a dusty road' and is a characteristic feature of chronic arsenic intoxication.

Investigations. Urinary excretion of more than 50 µg/L of arsenic in 24 hours is diagnostic of arsenic toxicity.

Management. Acute arsenic poisoning can be treated with the chelating agent dimercaprol. Topical application of keratolytic and

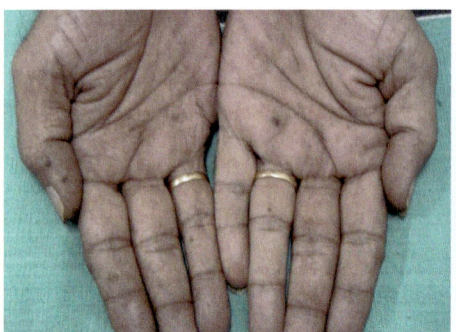
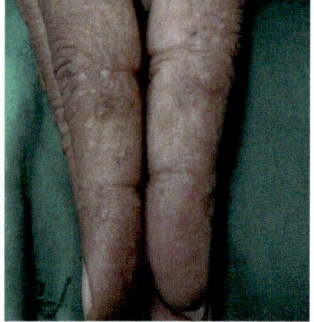

Figure 4.14 Arsenical keratosis.

retinoic acid creams may help to reduce skin lesions. Long-term oral retinoids (acitretin) may prevent malignant transformation of arsenical keratoses. Development of an erythematous halo around a papule may be an early indicator of malignant transformation and such papules should be excised.

4.15 Exogenous ochronosis

Exogenous ochronosis (EO) is caused by excessive use of hydroquinones in skin-whitening creams. The US Food and Drug Administration (FDA) has approved 4% hydroquinone cream for the treatment of melasma, freckles, senile lentigines, and hyperpigmentation. Though generally safe, adverse effects such as allergic contact dermatitis, dryness of nasolabial folds and infraorbital areas, erythema, stinging, and epidermal atrophy have all been recorded. EO is a chronic, recalcitrant, and rarer side effect. It was first described by Findlay in 1975 in patients who used inappropriate concentrations of hydroquinone of more than 6% over several years.[20]

Clinical presentation. EO is characterized by bluish-black hyperpigmentation (Figure 4.15). There are three clinical stages: initial erythema and mild pigmentation, black-colored milia and atrophy, and papulonodules. Once the third stage is reached the changes are permanent.

The putative mechanism of action causing these changes is that high levels of hydroquinone inhibit the enzyme homogentisic oxidase, resulting in the accumulation of homogentisic acid, which then polymerizes to form the ochronotic pigment. Sunlight worsens the condition.

Management. EO can be prevented by avoiding high concentrations of hydroquinone and using it for a shorter duration. The use of hydroquinone-containing creams should be terminated in patients with EO, and they should be advised on the regular use of sunscreens. Q-switched Alexandrite or Ruby laser therapy can be used to lighten the skin color.

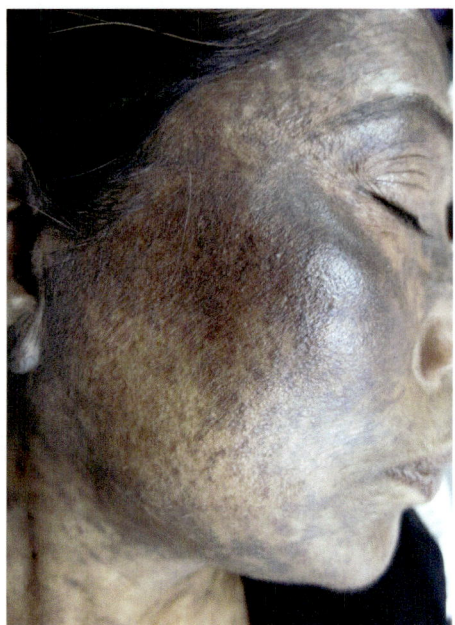

Figure 4.15 Exogenous ochronosis.

4.16 Confluent and reticulate papillomatosis

This is a rare form of papillomatosis. The cause is undetermined, but it has been variously regarded as a type of acanthosis nigricans, a genodermatosis, or an abnormal host response to *Malassezia* (*Pityrosporum*).[21]

Clinical presentation. Confluent and reticulate papillomatosis is the development of asymptomatic, slightly verrucous papules with a tendency to central confluence, forming a reticulate pattern in the periphery (Figure 4.16). The usual site of involvement is the upper part of the chest, back, neck, upper arm, and axillae.

There may be a familial tendency. Itching can occur with increasing environmental temperatures.

Histopathology shows hyperkeratosis, papillomatosis, and acanthosis. There may be hyperpigmentation of the basal layer. This is similar to acanthosis nigricans and epidermal nevus.

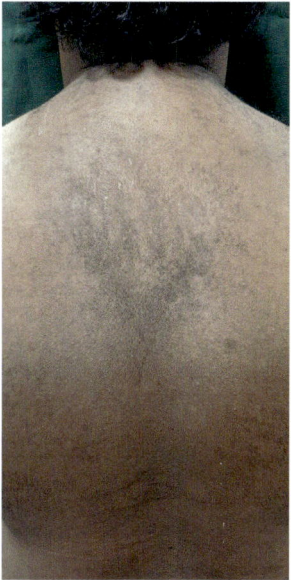

Figure 4.16 Confluent and reticulate papillomatosis.

Management. Confluent and reticulate papillomatosis responds to topical applications of selenium sulfide and other antifungals, but the treatment of choice is oral minocycline. The condition has also shown a limited response to calcipotriol and retinoids.

4.17 Tinea versicolor

Tinea versicolor is a superficial fungal infection caused by *Malassezia furfur*. It has low transmission rates.[22]

Clinical presentation. Tinea versicolor is mostly of cosmetic concern, although it may be itchy if patients get hot and sweaty. The chromic variety can mimic acanthosis nigricans and confluent and reticulated papillomatosis (Figure 4.17). The achromic variant simulates leprosy and post-kala-azar dermal leishmaniasis (PKDL).

Management. Both variants respond to topical and systemic antifungals but tend to recur, especially in summer.

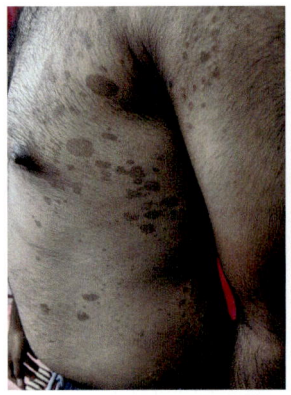
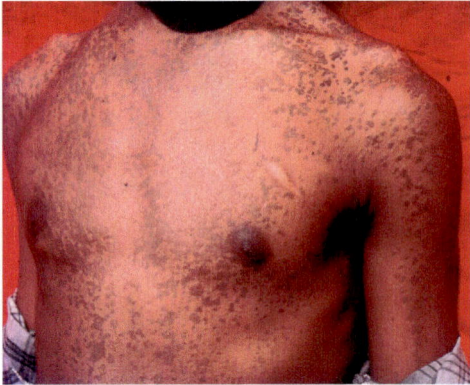

Figure 4.17 Chromic tinea versicolor.

4.18 Keloids

Keloids and hypertrophic scars are more common in SOC than white skin. Both occur in response to damage to the dermis. In keloids, the scar tissue extends beyond the site of trauma, while hypertrophic scars remain confined to the area of injury.[23] The exact etiology of keloids has not been ascertained but is known to involve abnormal collagen production and inadequate wound healing.

Clinical presentation. Early keloid lesions are mildly erythematous but older lesions are paler. The sites of predilection are the upper part of the back, deltoid region, presternal area, and earlobes, although they can occur elsewhere (Figure 4.18).

Predisposing factors for keloids include the patient's race and age, increased tension in the wound, and infection in the wound. Some keloids itch and others may be painful, but most are asymptomatic and only of cosmetic concern.

Management. As there is no satisfactory treatment for keloids, there should be an emphasis on prevention. Patients should be advised to avoid excessive movements that stretch the wound and should be shown how to keep the wound clean. Attempts to surgically remove a keloid may result in a bigger one at the same site. Intralesional steroids, intralesional bleomycin, and 5-fluorouracil have been

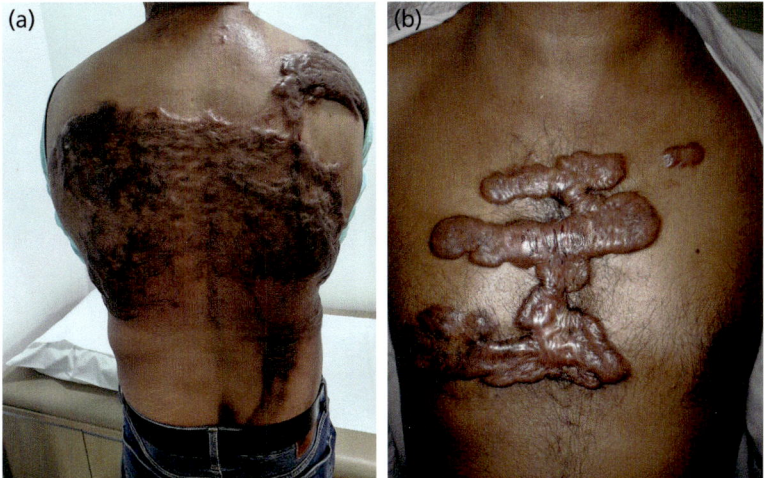

Figure 4.18 Extensive keloids on (a) back and (b) chest.

tried with some success. There are anecdotal reports for the use of cryotherapy and laser therapy, but as a rule there is no cure for keloids.

4.19 Post-kala-azar dermal leishmaniasis

Kala-azar (visceral leishmaniasis) was once endemic in several states in India, but following the eradication of the sandfly vector it has now become a rarity. Nevertheless, PKDL continues to present in dermatology clinics on rare occasions.[24] The disease is important from an epidemiological perspective. If the sandfly is introduced into a population with leishmaniasis, kala-azar may become endemic.

Clinical presentation. The skin lesions of PKDL appear about 6 months to 2 years after treatment of kala-azar. Nodules of various sizes present on the face, axillary folds, elbows, and knuckles (Figure 4.19), and are associated with hypopigmented macules on the trunk.

In a few patients of lighter complexion, a butterfly erythema may be visible on the face. Mucous membrane involvement is rarely seen. The patient's health is otherwise unaffected. The skin lesions' close resemblance to leprosy can lead to stigmatization of patients.

Histopathology. Slit smears from the nodules and from the hypopigmented macules show small spheres (2–5 µm in length) called

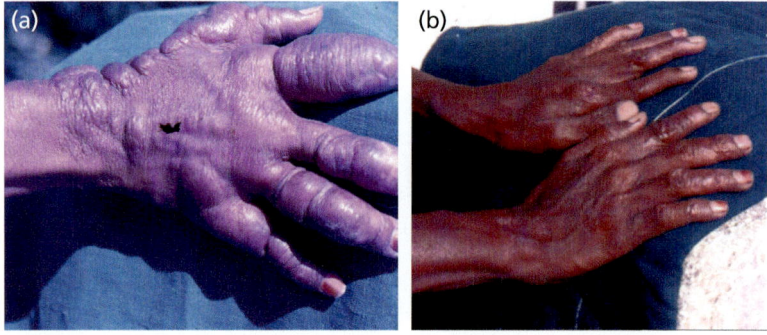

Figure 4.19 Post-kala-azar dermal leishmaniasis (PKDL) (a) before and (b) after treatment. This was the first patient with PKDL in the world to be treated with intravenous amphotericin, reported by Professor P Yesudian and Professor AS Thambiah.[25]

Leishman–Donovan bodies. These are the unflagellated form of the causative organism, the parasitic protozoan *Leishmania donovani*.

Management. The treatment of choice is oral miltefosine, 2.5 mg/kg/day, for 30–60 days. Previously, intramuscular sodium antimony gluconate, 200 mg on alternate days, was used. The resolution of the nodules can be assisted by oral potassium iodide, 1.8 g/day. Intravenous amphotericin B has been shown to be effective in a few recalcitrant cases compared with other modalities.

4.20 Physiological melanonychia striata

Physiological melanonychia striata is more prevalent in people of color than white-skinned people. It can present in individuals of all ages and affects both sexes equally.[26]

Clinical presentation. Physiological melanonychia striata is a tan, brown, or black streak within the nail (Figure 4.20). It is caused by increased activity of melanocytes or melanocytic hyperplasia in the nail matrix, which results in deposition of melanin in the nail plate. In the vast majority of cases, it is a benign condition. Rarely, however, an underlying malignant melanoma of the nail apparatus or subungual region may be a cause (Table 4.1).

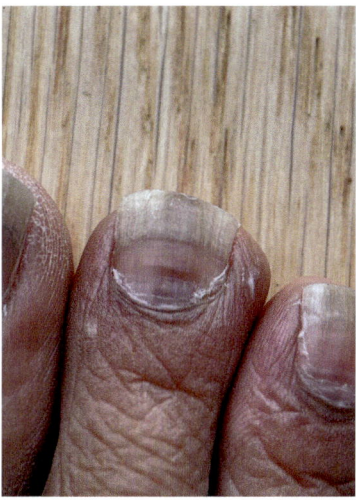

Figure 4.20 Physiological melanonychia striata.

TABLE 4.1

Features that should raise suspicion of subungual malignant melanoma in people with melanonychia striata

- Abrupt onset after middle age
- Family history of melanoma
- Rapid growth
- Darkening of a melanonychial band
- Pigment variation
- Blurry lateral borders
- Irregular elevation of the surface
- Band width >3 mm
- Proximal widening
- Dystrophy of affected nail
- Single rather than multiple nail involvement
- Periungual spread of pigmentation to adjacent cuticle
- Proximal and lateral nail folds (Hutchinson's sign)*

*Not pathognomonic for a nail apparatus melanoma.

It should be noted that Hutchinson's sign is not pathognomonic for subungual melanoma since it may be seen on one-third of nail lentigines or nail matrix nevi. It can also be seen in people with dark skin who have ethnic melanonychia, those with Laugier–Hunziker syndrome, Peutz–Jeghers syndrome, or Addison's disease, and after treatment with drugs, especially minocycline, biologics, and anticancer medications. In such cases, it is referred to as pseudo-Hutchinson's sign (see page 47).

Management. Biopsy is essential if a melanoma is suspected. Otherwise, reassurance will suffice.

4.21 Creeping eruptions in the skin

Cutaneous creeping eruptions are caused by the larvae of worms and flies moving in the skin. The larvae enter the body through direct contact with the skin, often from eggs deposited in the soil in animal feces.[27] Another unique form of creeping eruption can be caused by hair shafts or fragments embedded in the skin that migrate in a straight line.[28]

Clinical presentation. Symptoms of a parasitic creeping eruption include blisters, itching, and raised serpiginous tracks. The most common is cutaneous larva migrans, caused by the human hookworm *Ancylostoma duodenale* (Figure 4.21; also see Figures 1.17 and 2.4). It is usually the result of a single larva, though rarely large numbers of larvae may be found. The larvae move slowly within the epidermis at the rate of a few millimeters a day.

Cutaneous larva currens (racing) is caused by the larva of the threadworm *Strongyloides stercoralis*. It moves at a rate of several centimeters per hour within the upper dermis where there is less resistance than the epidermis.

The larva of the nematode *Dirofilaria repens* moves slowly, manifesting as a winding track under the skin or subcutaneous granulomas. The larvae of some fly species, such as *Gasterophilus* and *Hypoderma*, also move in the skin. They may be associated with Löffler's syndrome, a type of eosinophilic pneumonia.

Cutaneous pili migrans is when hair embedded in the stratum corneum is moved by biomechanical forces. Although it is rare in

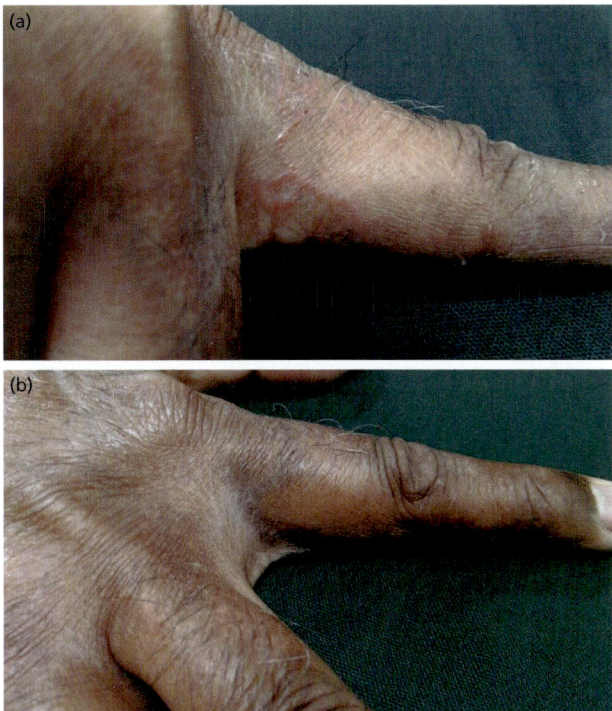

Figure 4.21 Larva migrans (a) in the finger web space of an avid gardener, (b) which resolved after treatment with albendazole.

children, it is reported on the soles of the feet as they walk on sharp hair fragments on the floor. In adults, it may occur in any frictional area, including the breast, abdomen, and neck. It mostly occurs in Asian people whose hairs are of larger diameter with stronger tensile strength. Movement of the black hair-like line causes erythema and it may be mistaken for cutaneous larva migrans. However, the hair moves in a straight line, unlike the tortuous tract of larva migrans.

Management of cutaneous pili migrans involves the daily application of 40% urea cream for a week to move the hair superficially so that it can be physically removed. Parasitic creeping eruptions may be treated with oral or topical anthelmintics, such as albendazole, thiabendazole, mebendazole, and ivermectin.

Key points – presentation and management of dermatoses predominantly seen in skin of color

- There are several dermatoses that are unique to, or more prevalent in, people with SOC.
- Early-stage MF, a form of CTCL, tends to go undetected or is misdiagnosed in SOC; earlier recognition may improve outcomes.
- Pigmentary disorders are generally more common in individuals with SOC.
- Patients with follicular and scarring disorders, which tend to disproportionately affect individuals with SOC, often present for cosmetic reasons. These dermatoses cause emotional distress and stigmatization, reducing quality of life.

References

1. Hinds GA, Heald P. Cutaneous T-cell lymphoma in skin of color. *J Am Acad Dermatol*. 2009;60(3):359-375.
2. Huang AH, Kwatra SG, Khanna R, Semenov YR, Okoye GA, Sweren RJ. Racial disparities in the clinical presentation and prognosis of patients with mycosis fungoides. *J Natl Med Assoc*. 2019;111(6):633-639.
3. Espinosa ML, Walker CJ, Guitart J, Mhlaba JM. Morphology of mycosis fungoides and Sézary syndrome in skin of color. *Cutis*. 2022;109(3):E3-E7.
4. Alimi Y, Iwanaga J, Loukas M, et al. A comprehensive review of Mongolian spots with an update on atypical presentations. *Childs Nerv Syst*. 2018;34(12):2371-2376.
5. Cordova A. The Mongolian spot: a study of ethnic differences and a literature review. *Clin Pediatr (Phila)*. 1981;20(11):714-719.
6. Gupta D, Thappa DM. Dermatoses due to Indian cultural practices. *Indian J Dermatol*. 2015;60(1):3-12.
7. Maghfour J, Ogunleye T. A systematic review on the treatment of dermatosis papulosa nigra. *J Drugs Dermatol*. 2021;20(4):467-472.

8. Kaimal S, D'Souza M, Kumari R. Dermatitis cruris pustulosa et atrophicans. *Indian J Dermatol Venereol Leprol.* 2009;75(4):348-355.
9. Sharma VK, Sethuraman G. Parthenium dermatitis. *Dermatitis.* 2007;18(4):183-190.
10. Malhotra AK, Lis JA, Ramam M. Cydnidae (burrowing bug) pigmentation: a novel arthropod dermatosis. *JAMA Dermatol.* 2015;151(2):232-233.
11. Ogunbiyi A. Pseudofolliculitis barbae; current treatment options. *Clin Cosmet Investig Dermatol.* 2019;12:241-247.
12. Bandhlish A, Aggarwal A, Koranne RV. A clinico-epidemiological study of macular amyloidosis from North India. *Indian J Dermatol.* 2012;57(4):269-274.
13. Robles-Méndez JC, Rizo-Frías P, Herz-Ruelas ME, Pandya AG, Ocampo Candiani J. Lichen planus pigmentosus and its variants: review and update. *Int J Dermatol.* 2018;57(5):505-514.
14. Sarkar R, Vinay K, Bishnoi A, et al. A Delphi consensus on the nomenclature and diagnosis of lichen planus pigmentosus and related entities. *Indian J Dermatol Venereol Leprol.* 2023;89(1):41-46.
15. Weston G, Payette M. Update on lichen planus and its clinical variants. *Int J Womens Dermatol.* 2015;1(3):140-149.
16. Vashi NA, Kundu RV. Facial hyperpigmentation: causes and treatment. *Br J Dermatol.* 2013;169(Suppl 3):41-56.
17. Sonthalia S, Agrawal M, Sharma P, Pandey A. Maturational hyperpigmentation: cutaneous marker of metabolic syndrome. *Dermatol Pract Concept.* 2020;10(2):e2020046.
18. Nair SP, Gomathy M, Kumar GN. Disseminate and recurrent infundibulofolliculitis in an Indian patient: a case report with review of literature. *Indian Dermatol Online J.* 2017;8(1):39-41.
19. Shajil C, Mahabal GD. Arsenical keratosis. In: *StatPearls.* StatPearls Publishing; 2023. Last accessed 1 May 2023. ncbi.nlm.nih.gov/books/NBK560570
20. Bhattar PA, Zawar VP, Godse KV, Patil SP, Nadkarni NJ, Gautam MM. Exogenous ochronosis. *Indian J Dermatol.* 2015;60(6):537-543.
21. Le C, Bedocs PM. Confluent and reticulated papillomatosis. In: *StatPearls.* StatPearls Publishing; 2023. Last accessed 1 May 2023. ncbi.nlm.nih.gov/books/NBK459130
22. Karray M, McKinney WP. Tinea versicolor. In: *StatPearls.* StatPearls Publishing; 2023. Last accessed 1 May 2023. ncbi.nlm.nih.gov/books/NBK482500
23. Betarbet U, Blalock TW. Keloids: a review of etiology, prevention, and treatment. *J Clin Aesthet Dermatol.* 2020;13(2):33-43.
24. Zijlstra EE, Musa AM, Khalil EAG, el-Hassan IM, el-Hassan AM. Post-kala-azar dermal leishmaniasis. *Lancet Infect Dis.* 2003;3(2):87-98.

25. Yesudian P, Thambiah AS. Amphotericin B therapy in dermal leishmanoid. *Arch Dermatol.* 1974;109(5): 720-722.
26. Singal A, Bisherwal K. Melanonychia: etiology, diagnosis, and treatment. *Indian Dermatol Online J.* 2020;11(1):1-11.
27. Maxfield L, Crane JS. Cutaneous larva migrans. In: *StatPearls.* StatPearls Publishing; 2023. Last accessed 10 May 2023. ncbi.nlm.nih.gov/books/ NBK507706
28. Kim YJ, Kim JI, Hwang SH, et al. Cutaneous pili migrans. *Ann Dermatol.* 2014;26(4):534-535.

Useful resources

American Academy of Dermatology
aad.org

American Skin Association
americanskin.org

British Association of Dermatologists
bad.org.uk

British Skin Foundation
britishskinfoundation.org.uk

DermNet – dermatological conditions in skin of colour
dermnetnz.org/topics/skin-conditions-in-skin-of-colour

European Academy of Dermatology & Venereology
eadv.org

Global Vitiligo Foundation
globalvitiligofoundation.org

Indian Association of Dermatologists, Venereologists and Leprologists
iadvl.org

International League of Dermatological Societies
ilds.org

Keloid Research Foundation
keloidresearchfoundation.org

Pigmentary Disorders Society
pigmentarydisorderssociety.com

Primary Care Dermatology Society (UK)
pcds.org.uk

Skin of Color Society
skinofcolorsociety.org

Skin Deep
dftbskindeep.com

Skin Inflammation & Psoriasis International Network
spindermatology.org

Index

acne *41*, 72–4
acneiform dermatoses 40–1
actinic lichen planus 106, *107*
adalimumab 77, 79
adapalene 72
Addison's disease *18*
allergic contact dermatitis
 kumkum 97
 Parthenium weed 99–101
 patch testing 59, 67, *68*
amphotericin B 116
amyloidosis, macular 103–4
annular lesions 29–30
anthelmintics 119
antibiotics 73, 78–9, 99, 102, 113
antifungal agents 113, 116
arsenical keratosis *82*, 110–11
atopic dermatitis (eczema) *62*, 74–6
 post-treatment 76
bacterial infections 12, 58, 60
 bullous impetigo *24*
 DCPA 98–9
 syphilis 60
basal cell carcinoma (BCC) 82–3
bindi-induced dermatitis 96–7
biological treatments 76, 77, 79
biopsy 59, 82, 85

blaschkoid dermatoses *17*, 35–6
bleomycin reaction *19*
blisters, infantile 23–5
blood tests 58–9, 60–2
Bowen's disease 82
bullous dermatoses 23–5
bullous impetigo *24*

calcineurin inhibitors 76, 104
cancer 81
 BCC 82–3
 detection 59, 85, 111
 Kaposi's sarcoma *20*
 melanoma 59, 84–5, 117
 mycosis fungoides *32*, 94–5
 prevention 85–7
 SCC 81–2
causes 10–52
children
 dermal melanocytosis 95–6
 infantile blisters 23–5
 photosensitive disorders 43–4
Christmas-tree pattern 33–4
chromoblastomycosis *23*
ciclosporin 76
clinical presentation 10–52
 acne *41*, 72, *73*
 arsenical keratosis *82*, 110
 BCC 83
 confluent and reticulate papillomatosis 112, *113*

creeping eruptions *28*, 30, *63*, 118–19
Cydnidae pigmentation 101–2
DCPA 98–9
dermal melanocytosis 95, *96*
dermatosis papulosa nigra 97–8
disseminated infundibulofolliculitis 109
eczema *62*, 74–5
EO 111, *112*
HS *22*, 78, *79*
keloids 114, *115*
larva migrans *28*, 30, *63*, 118, *119*
lichen planus *31*, 105, 106, *107*
macular amyloidosis 103–4
maturational hyperpigmentation 107–8
melanoma 84–5, 117
melanonychia striata 116–18
mycosis fungoides *32*, 94, *95*
Parthenium dermatitis 100
PFB 102, *103*
PIH 72, 80
PKDL *44*, 115–16
psoriasis 25, 29, 40, 50, 61, 77
SCC 82
 tinea versicolor 113, *114*
comedones 22, 72
confluent and reticulate papillomatosis 112–13

125

creeping eruptions 118–19
larva migrans 28, 30, 63, 118, *119*
cutaneous pili migrans 118–19
Cydnidae pigmentation 101–2

Darier's disease *51*
Demodex folliculitis *41*
dermal melanocytosis 95–6
dermatitis cruris pustulosa et atrophicans (DCPA) 98–9
dermatitis herpetiformis *11*
dermatoscopy 59, 102
dermatosis papulosa nigra 97–8
diabetes mellitus *38*, 107
diagnosis 10, 58
digitate dermatoses 32–3
dimercaprol 110
disseminated infundibulofolliculitis 109
distribution patterns 30–6
drug reactions *19*, *39*

ears, thickened pinnae 46–7
eczema 62, 74–6
  post-treatment *76*
eosinophilia 61–3
eosinophilic spongiosis 63
epidermal nevus *36*
erythema ab igne *19*
etiology 10–52
eumycetoma 65
exogenous ochronosis (EO) 111, *112*

eyebrows, partial loss 46

facial dermatoses
  acne *41*, 72–4
  contact dermatitis 97, *100*
  dermatosis papulosa nigra 98
  destructive nasal lesions 45
  eyebrow partial loss 46
  leonine facies 44–5
  LPP *105*
  maturational hyperpigmentation 107–8
  melasma 87–8
  PFB 102–3
  thickened pinnae 46–7
  white patches 16–17, *89*
feet
  Cydnidae bug secretions 101–2
  eumycetoma 65
  plantar pustules 26–7
fever and rash 13–14
folliculitis 40
  DCPA 98–9
  disseminated infundibulofolliculitis 109
  post-transplant *41*
fungal infections
  chromoblastomycosis 23
  eumycetoma 65
  histoplasmosis 64
  investigations 58, 65
  sporotrichosis 34
  tinea versicolor 113, *114*
granuloma, infectious 63–5

hair
  cutaneous pili migrans 118–19

hair *(contd)*
  PFB 102–3
  tests 58
hair dye reactions 68, 87, 104
hands *see* nails; palms
hidradenitis suppurativa (HS) 22, 78–80, 89
histopathology 63–7, 96, 99, 104, 105, 108, 109, 112, 115–16
histoplasmosis 64
hookworm (larva migrans) 28, 30, 63, 118, *119*
Hutchinson's sign 118
hydroquinone 81, 111
hyperhidrosis 11–13
hyperkeratotic psoriasis 40
hyperpigmentation
  EO 111, *112*
  generalized 14–15
  LPP 104–6
  maturational 107–8
  melasma 87–8
  palmar 18–19
  post-inflammatory 72, 80–1
hypertrophic scars 114
hypopigmentation
  on face 16–17
  hair dye use 87
  linear 17–18
  vitiligo 88, *89*

imaging 59
imatinib reaction *39*
infantile blisters 23–5
infections
  granulomas 63–5
  tests 58, 60
  see also specific disorders
interleukin inhibitors 76, 77, 79
investigations 58–69, 99, 110

Index

isotretinoin 73
itching without rash 10–11

Janus kinase inhibitors 76

kala-azar (PKDL) 44, 115–16
Kaposi's sarcoma 20
keloids 114–15
koilonychia 48–9
kumkum-induced dermatitis 96–7
Kyrle's disease 38

larva currens 118
larva migrans 28, 30, 63, 118, 119
laser therapy 73–4, 81, 96, 111
leishmaniasis 44, 65, 115–16
leonine facies 44–5
leprosy 58, 65
lichen nitidus 39
lichen planus
  actinic (ALP) 106, 107
  linear 31
  pigmentosus (LPP) 104–6
lichen striatus 17
lichenoid dermatoses 38–9
linear morphology 17–18, 31–2
lipoid proteinosis 42, 47
lupus vulgaris 12

macular amyloidosis 103–4
malignancy *see* cancer
maturational hyperpigmentation 107–8
melanoma 59, 84–5, 117

melanonychia striata 116–18
melasma 87–8
methotrexate 77
migratory dermatoses 30–1
  see also creeping eruptions
miltefosine 116
moisturizers 75
Mongolian blue spot 95–6
mpox 27
morphea (en coup de sabre) 31
mycosis fungoides 32, 94–5

nail clippings 58
nails
  koilonychia 48–9
  melanonychia striata 116–18
  pitting 49–50
  pseudo-Hutchinson sign 47–8, 118
nasal lesions 45
neoplasms *see* cancer
neurofibroma 21
neurofibromatosis 15

oral pigmentation 20–1

Paederus dermatitis 31
palms
  Addison's disease 18
  arsenical keratosis 82, 110–11
  hyperpigmentation 18–19
  maculopapular rash (syphilis) 60
  pits 50–1
  pustules 26–7
paraphenylenediamine reaction 68, 104

parasitic infections 118
  Demodex folliculitis 41
  larva migrans 28, 30, 63, 118, 119
  leishmaniasis 44, 65, 115–16
Parthenium dermatitis 99–101
patch testing 59, 67, 68
pathergy 36–7
peels 81
pellagra-like dermatoses 41–2
perforating disorders 37–8
photoprotection 80, 85–7
photosensitive disorders in children 43–4
phototherapy 76, 77, 94
pigmentation
  Cydnidae bug secretions 101–2
  macular amyloidosis 103–4
  oral 20–1
  peri/subungual 47–8, 116–18
  and psychosocial distress 87–9
  reticulate acropigmentation 19–20
  tumors 21
  see also hyperpigmentation; hypopigmentation
pitted nails 49–50
pitted palms 50–1
pityriasis rosea-like eruption 33–4
plantar dermatoses
  Cydnidae bug secretions 101–2
  pustules 26–7
polycystic ovary syndrome 72, 79
polymorphic light eruption 16, 43

post-inflammatory hyperpigmentation (PIH) 72, 80–1
post-kala-azar dermal leishmaniasis (PKDL) *44*, 115–16
post-viral infection *26*
presentation *see* clinical presentation
prurigo nodularis *66*
pruritis without rash 10–11
pseudo-Hutchinson sign 47–8, 118
pseudoepitheliomatous hyperplasia 66–7
pseudofolliculitis barbae (PFB) 102–3
psoriasiform dermatoses 39–40
psoriasis 77, 89
  hyperkeratotic *40*
  nail pitting *50*
  plaque *29*, *40*
  post-treatment 78
  pustular *25*
  vitamin D deficiency *61*
psychological distress 87–9
pustular psoriasis *25*
pustules
  palmoplantar 26–7
  sterile 25–6
pyoderma gangrenosum *37*
pyrexia and rash 13–14

rashes
  annular 29–30

rashes *(contd)*
  Christmas-tree 33–4
  with fever 13–14
  migratory 30
  syphilis *60*
reticulate acropigmentation 19–20
retinoids 72, 73, 81, 111

scarring
  acne 73–4
  keloids 114–15
scrapings 58
self-examination (for cancer) 85
serpiginous lesions 28
shaving 102–3
skin lightening 7–8, 72
  EO 111, *112*
slit skin smears 58, 115–16
spironolactone 73
Splendore-Hoeppli phenomenon 65–6
sporotrichoid distribution 34–5
squamous cell carcinoma (SCC) 81–2
steroids 73, 75, 79, 104, 106
subungual pigmentation 47–8, 118
sunscreen 80, 85–6
swabs 58
sweating, excessive 11–13
symptoms *see* clinical presentation
syphilis *60*

systemic lupus erythematosus (SLE) *14*

tazarotene 72
tests 58–69, 110
threadworm 118
tinea versicolor 113, *114*
TNFα inhibitors 77, 79
trichoepithelioma *21*
trigeminal trophic syndrome *45*
tuberculosis 12
tumors
  benign *15*, *21*, *27*
  malignant *see* cancer

umbilicated lesions *27*
urinalysis 110

varioliform scarring 42–3
VDRL test 60–1
verrucous dermatoses 22–3
viral infections *27*, 58
vitamin B3 deficiency (pellagra) 41, *42*
vitamin D deficiency 61
vitiligo 88, *89*

warty dermatoses 22–3
white patches *see* hypopigmentation
Wood's light examination 59

zosteriform dermatoses 35–6